First International Moxifloxacin Symposium – Berlin, 1999

Springer
Berlin
Heidelberg
New York
Barcelona
Hong Kong
London
Milan
Paris
Singapore
Tokyo

L. MANDELL (ED.)

First International Moxifloxacin Symposium
Berlin, 1999

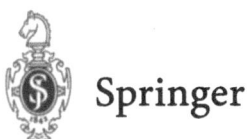 Springer

PROF. LIONEL MANDELL

McMaster University
Division of Infectious Diseases
Henderson General Hospital
711 Concession Street
Hamilton, Ontario L8V1C3
Canada

ISBN-13:978-3-642-64081-0   Springer-Verlag Berlin Heidelberg New York

Die Deutsche Bibliothek – CIP-Einheitsaufnahme

International Moxifloxacin Symposium <1, 1999, Berlin>:
Proceedings of the First International Moxifloxacin Symposium / L.
Mandell (ed.). – Berlin ; Heidelberg ; New York ; Barcelona ;
Hongkong ; London ; Milan ; Paris ; Singapore ; Tokyo : Springer,
1999
   ISBN-13:978-3-642-64081-0   e-ISBN-13:978-3-642-59681-0
   DOI: 10.1007/978-3-642-59681-0

Cover design: Design & Production GmbH, Heidelberg
Typesetting: Fotosatz-Service Köhler GmbH, 97084 Würzburg

SPIN: 10742010   18/3134 – 5 4 3 2 1 0 – Printed on acid-free paper

Preface

The 1st International Moxifloxacin symposium took place in Berlin Germany February 18–20, 1999. The purpose of this meeting was to introduce the medical and scientific communities to this exciting new fluoroquinolone and to define its role in the management of respiratory tract infections. The fluoroquinolones as a class are an important part of our therapeutic armamentarium and moxifloxacin is a unique addition to this class of compounds.

This symposium brought together physician/scientists from around the world to present and discuss the moxifloxacin data. The information from this important meeting are presented in these proceedings and are organized under the following headings:

Part I   Antimicrobial chemotherapy
Part II   Pre-clinical microbiology
Part III Pharmacology
Part IV   Clinical needs in the millennium
Part V   Round table discussion

The modifications to the basic quinolone structure resulting in moxifloxacin have produced a drug with unique in vitro, and pharmacokinetic/pharmaco-dynamic properties. The drug has a very broad spectrum of antimicrobial activity, is well absorbed and can be taken only once daily. Its profile makes it an excellent therapeutic option for many types of respiratory tract infections.

It is hoped that our clinical and laboratory colleagues will be as excited by this data as we are and we look forward to further work with this unique and interesting compound.

L. MANDELL

Table of Contents

Introduction to the Symposium 1
LIONEL MANDELL

PART 1 – Antimicrobial Chemotherapy

Antimicrobial Chemotherapy – Today 7
JOHN DAVID WILLIAMS

Antimicrobial Chemotherapy – Tomorrow 12
HARTMUT LODE

PART 2 – Pre-clinical

Pre-clinical Microbiology – Streptococcus Pneumoniae 21
REGINE HAKENBECK

Pre-clinical Microbiology – Gram-positive Cocci 27
SILVANO ESPOSITO

Pre-clinical Microbiology – Atypical Organisms 31
CÉCILE M. BÉBÉAR

Pre-clinical Microbiology – Summary I 36
BERND WIEDEMANN

Pre-clinical Microbiology – Mycobacteria 37
STEPHEN H. GILLESPIE

In-vitro Activity of Moxifloxacin [Bay 12-8039], an 8-methoxy Quinolone,
Compared to Other Fluoroquinolones Against Anaerobic Bacteria 43
ELLIE GOLDSTEIN

Pre-clinical Microbiology – Fastidious Gram-negative Bacteria 49
ADOLF BAUERNFEIND

Pre-clinical Microbiology – Respiratory Tract Infections
Susceptibility Survey – USA 54
DANIEL SAHM

Pre-clinical Microbiology – Respiratory Tract Infections
Susceptibility Survey – Europe 59
DAVID FELMINGHAM

Pre-clinical Microbiology – Respiratory Tract Infections
Susceptibility Survey – Japan 67
KAZUNORI TOMONO

Mechanisms of Fluoroquinolone Action and Resistance 75
KARL DRLICA

Pre-clinical Microbiology – Summary II 84
BERND WIEDEMANN

PART 3 – Pharmacology

Pharmacokinetics and Pharmacodynamics of Antimicrobials 89
RICHARD WISE

Mini-Reviews – Pharmacokinetics/Pharmacodynamics (PK/PD) 94
JEROME J. SCHENTAG

In vitro Models as Predictors of the Antimicrobial Effect of Moxifloxacin
and Other Fluoroquinolones 98
STEPHEN ZINNER

In vitro Models of Infection – Pharmacokinetic/Pharmacodynamic
Correlates 104
ALASDAIR P. MCGOWAN

Animal Model Experiences with Moxifloxacin 111
JAMES M. STECKELBERG

Current Thinking About Pharmacokinetics and Pharmacodynamics
of Antimicrobials 118
JOHN TURNIDGE

Pharmacology of Moxifloxacin – Absorption, Distribution, Metabolism
and Excretion 122
CARL ERIK NORD

Antimicrobial Drug-Drug Interations – Focus on Fluoroquinolones 127
GARY E. STEIN

Pharmacology – Tissue Distribution 130
ETHAN RUBINSTEIN

Fluoroquinolones Phototoxicity – Moxifloxacin in Context 134
JAMES FERGUSON

Fluoroquinolone Safety and Tolerability 138
PETER BALL

PART 4 – Clinical Needs in the Millenium

Clinical Needs in the Millenium – Community Acquired Pneumonia . . . 147
PAUL LÉOPHONTE

Clinical Needs in the Millenium – Pneumonia – The Role of Moxifloxacin   154
MARTIN SPRINGSKLEE

Clinical Needs in the Millenium – Acute Exacerbations
of Chronic Bronchitis 159
ROBERT WILSON

Clinical Needs in the Millenium – Acute Exacerbations
of Chronic Bronchitis – The Role of Moxifloxacin 165
DEBORAH CHURCH

Clinical Needs in the Millenium – Rhinosinusitis 170
VALERIE J. LUND

Clinical Needs in the Millenium – Rhinosinusitis –
The Role of Moxifloxacin 175
BARBARA HAMPEL

Discussion on Clinical Needs in the Millenium 179

PART 5 – Round Table Discussion

Round Table Discussion – Introduction 185

Round Table Discussion – Hospital Issues 186

Round Table Discussion – Community Issues 191

List of contributors

PETER BALL
6 Gilchrist Row
KY 16 8XU St. Andrews Fife,
Scotland, United Kingdom

ADOLF BAUERNFEIND
Ludwig-Maximilians-Universität
Pettenkofer-Institut of Hygiene
und med. Mikrobiologie
Pettenkoferstraße 9 a
80336 Munich, Germany

CÉCILE M. BÉBÉAR
Laboratoire de Bactériologie,
Université Bordeaux 2
146 rue Léo Saignat
33076 Bordeaux Cedex, France

DEBORAH CHURCH
Bayer Corporation
Medical Department
400 Morgan Lane
06516 West Haven, Conneticut, USA

KARL DRLICA
Public Health Research Institute
455 First Avenue
100016 New York, New York, USA

SILVANO ESPOSITO
Clinica Malattie Infettive
Seconda Università
degli Studi di Napoli
Facoltà di Medicina
Ospedale Gesù e Maria
Via D. Cotugno 1
80135 Napoli, Italy

DAVID FELMINGHAM
G. R. Micro Ltd.
7–9 William Road
NW1 3ER London, United Kingdom

JAMES FERGUSON
Photobiology Unit
Dermatology Department
Ninewells Hospital
and Medical School
University of Dundee
Dundee, Scotland DD1 9SY
United Kingdom

STEPHEN H. GILLESPIE
Royal Free and University Hospital
College Medical School
Department of Medical Microbiology
University College London
Royal Free Campus
Rowland Hill Street
NW3 2PF London, United Kingdom

ELLIE J. C. GOLDSTEIN
2021 Santa Monica Blvd
Suite 640 E
90404-2208 Santa Monica,
California, USA

BARBARA HAMPEL
Euro CPL for Moxifloxacin
BAYER Vital GmbH & Co. KG
BV-PH-MED Klifo AI
Building D 162
51368 Leverkusen, Germany

REGINE HAKENBECK
Universität Kaiserslautern
Fachbereich Biologie
Abl-Mikrobiologie
Postfach 3049
67653 Kaiserslautern, Germay

PAUL LÉOPHONTE
Service de Pneumologie
Université Paul Sabatier
Hôpital Tolouse-Rangueil
1, avenue J. Poulhès
31403 Toulouse, Cedex 4, France

HARTMUT LODE
Freie Universität Berlin
Chief, Chest and Infectious Disease
Department
City Hospital Zehlendorf-
Heckeshorn
14109 Berlin, Germany

VALERIE J. LUND
University College London
Medical School
Professional Unit
Royal National Throat Nose &
Ear Hospital
330/332 Gray's Inn Road
WC1X 8DA London,
United Kingdom

ALASDAIR P. MACGOWAN
Bristol Centre for Antimicrobial
Research Evaluation
Department of Medical Microbiology
Southmead Hospital
Westbody – on – Trym
BS10 5NB Bristol, United Kingdom

LIONEL A. MANDELL
McMaster University
Division of Infectious Diseases
Henderson General Hospital
711 Concession Street
L8V 1C3 Hamilton, Ontario,
Canada

CARL ERIK NORD
Department of Immunology,
Microbiology, Pathology &
Infectious Diseases
Huddinge University Hospital
141 86 Huddinge, Sweden

ETHAN RUBINSTEIN
Infectious Diseases Unit
Chaim Sheba Medical Center
52621 Tel-Hashomer, Israel

DANIEL SAHM
MRL Pharmaceutical Services, Inc.
136654 Dulles Technology Drive,
Suite 200
20171 Herndon, Virginia, USA

JEROME J. SCHENTAG
Millard Fillmore Hospital
Clinical Pharmacokinetics Unit
3 Gates Circle
14209 Buffalo, New York, USA

MARTIN SPRINGSKLEE
Bayer AG
Business Group Pharma
Product Development
SPM Moxifloxacin
42096 Wuppertal, Germany

JAMES STECKELBERG
Mayo Clinic
200 First Street, SW
55905 Rochester, Minesota, USA

GARY E. STEIN
Michigan State University
B320 Life Sciences Building
48824 East Lansing, Michigan, USA

KAZUNORI TOMONO
Department of Internal Medicine II
Nagasaki University School
of Medicine
Sakomoto 1-7-1
852-8501 Nagasaki, Japan

JOHN TURNIDGE
Department of Microbiology
and Infectious Diseases
Women's & Children's Hospital
72 King William Road
5006 North Adelaide, South Australia,
Australia

BERND WIEDEMANN
University of Bonn
Pharmaceutical Microbiology
Meckenheimer Allee 168
53115 Bonn, Germany

JOHN DAVID WILLIAMS
7 William Road
NW1 3ER Londeon,
United Kingdom

ROBERT WILSON
Imperial College School of Medicine
Host Defence Unit
National Heart & Lung Institute
Emmanuel Kaye Building
Manresa Road
SW3 6LR London, United Kingdom

RICHARD WISE
Department of Medical Microbiology
City Hospital NHS Trust
Dudley Road
B18 7QH Birmingham, United Kingdom

STEPHEN ZINNER
Mount Auburn Hospital
330 Mount Auburn Road
MA 02138 Cambridge, United States

CHAPTER 1

Introduction to the Symposium

LIONEL MANDELL

This symposium, "The Idea Realized", was conceived to illustrate how drug design has become a reality. Data presented at this symposium cover the in-vitro activity of moxifloxacin, its mode of action, pharmacology, pharmacokinetics, pharmacodynamics, clinical efficacy and tolerability.

Although the clinical relevance of penicillin resistance among isolates of *Streptococcus pneumoniae* can be debated, there is no question that this resistance can be documented *in vitro*. Results of testing at 180 clinical centres across the United States between January 1st and October 31st, 1998 are summarised in Table 1 [1]. Of the pneumococcal blood isolates, 72.5% were sensitive and the remainder showed reduced susceptibility to penicillin, with a ratio of approximately 2:1 for intermediate to high level resistant organisms. Of the respiratory isolates, only one-half were susceptible, and there was a 1:1 ratio of intermediate to high level resistance to penicillin. It is disconcerting to note that not only has the percentage of intermediate and resistant isolates risen in recent years, but the ratio of intermediate to resistant strains has shifted from 3 or 4:1 to almost 1:1.

Of pneumococcal blood isolates that were penicillin-sensitive (pen-S), only 6% were resistant to macrolides, such as erythromycin. For those that were penicillin-resistant (pen-R), however, this figure jumped to 63%. Similarly, only 8% of pen-S respiratory isolates were resistant to erythromycin, while 67% of pen-R respiratory isolates showed erythromycin resistance. Literature reports of

Table 1. Characteristics of *Streptococcus pneumoniae* in 180 centres across U.S. (Jan 1/98 – Oct 31/98). S – susceptible, I – intermediate, R – resistant

Penicillin					Erythromycin	
Source	Total	% S	% I	% R	Source	% R
Blood	1693	72.5	18	9.5	*Blood*	
					Pen S.	5.7
					Pen R.	62.5
Respiratory	2500	50.4	27.4	22.2	*Respiratory*	
					Pen S.	8.3
					Pen R.	67.3

clinical macrolide failures may be difficult to find at this time, but these in vitro data sound a clear warning.

Several papers have investigated the impact of growing drug resistance using different outcome measures. Plouffe et al. [2] showed that hospitalised patients with community acquired pneumococcal pneumonia and bacteraemia, had their length of stay increased by 3.7 days compared to those with penicillin susceptible infection. Einnarson [3] showed similar results. With mortality as an outcome, it is commonly reported that Pallares et al. [4] showed no difference between susceptible and non-susceptible strains. However, the original analysis showed 38% mortality for penicillin non-susceptible versus 24% for penicillin-susceptible infected patients (p-value of 0.001). Further analysis to account for monomicrobial infections resulted in reported, mortality rates of 25% and 19%, respectively. A similar 6% difference was found by Einnarson et al., who found 11% versus 5% mortality rares for penicillin-resistant and penicillin susceptible strains respectively.

Resistance also results in rising drug costs. In 1995, the Office of Technology Assessment in the United States estimated the total annual direct cost of drug resistance to be $4 billion US [5] accounting for 0.5% of total U.S. health care costs for that year. Cost-effectiveness may be affected by increasing resistance in many ways. Less effective agents may be used in therapy, resulting in waste of precious health care dollars and there may be need for the implementation of improved surveillance systems to monitor emerging drug-resistance. More expensive drugs may be required to treat resistant infections and ineffective agents may result increased morbidity, mortality and length of hospital stay.

Community-acquired pneumonia (CAP) provides a good of bacterial resistance. However, the data do not back this up. They simply show the impact of CAP and not necessarily from resistance. Though it comprises only a small portion of all respiratory tract infections (approximately 10%), it is estimated that there are 3–4 million cases of CAP annually, resulting in approximately 600,000 cases being hospitalised, 64 million days of restricted activity, and 78,000 deaths per year in the U.S. Despite these figures, the general public and many physicians are unaware of the impact of this disease. This is all the more astounding when it is revealed that CAP is the most common cause of death from infection and, when compared to all causes of death in the United States (including heart attacks, cancer, etc...), it is the sixth most common cause overall [6, 7].

Yet things are changing and paradigms are shifting. The increase in resistance is fueling our need for new anti-infective agents. However, one of the obstacles in the search for these new compounds is the time required to reach develop then. It usually takes at least five years and requires an absolute minimum of $300 million US$ such time and resource commitments have often proven prohibitive in the past. Fortunately, knowledge of structure activity relationships, makes it possible to develop "designer drugs" and move the process along more rapidly and Bayer is a demonstrated leader in the use of this approach.

Given what is known about current resistance issues and clinical situations Bayer has constructed a 'wish list' for new anti-infectives. The desired properties include an excellent spectrum of activity with low induction of resistance. Ideally, the drug would have both oral and IV formulations and would display excellent pharmacokinetic and pharmacodynamic properties. Obviously the drug should be clinically effective and adverse drug reactions and drug interactions must be minimal. Finally, the drug must be cost effective.

Bayer has a long record of anti-infective research with experience in sulphonamides, penicillins, azoles and the fluoroquinolones. They have put this experience to use in the development of Bay 12-8039, a new fluoroquinolone known as moxifloxacin. Moxifloxacin was designed to fulfil some of the needs mentioned above. 1. to be active against resistant and atypical pathogens. 2. to permit once daily dosing in order to enhance compliance. 3. to achieve sufficient concentration at the site of infection 4. to be well tolerated and effective.

This has been one of the fastest development processes ever achieved. Moxifloxacin was discovered in 1990 and entered the clinical research phase in 1995. Phase I was completed in 7 months from August 1995 to February 1996 (610 patients). Phase II was initiated in June and completed in December of 1996, and Phase III began in November 1996 and was completed in June of 1998. Altogether 8418 patients were enrolled in Phase II and III studies, and it took only 3 years from the start of clinical development to regulatory submission.

It has been a pleasure to take part in this symposium and we hope that you will share our excitement when you read these papers.

References

1. Dr. Daniel Sahm, personal communication.
2. Plouffe JF, Breiman RF, Facklam RR (1996) Bacteremia with Streptococcus pneumoniae. Implications for therapy and prevention. Franklin County Pneumonia Study Group. Journal of the American Medical Association 275(3):194–198
3. Einarsson S, Kristjansson M, Kristinsson KG, Kjartansson G, Jonsson S (1998) Pneumonia caused by penicillin-non-susceptible and penicillin-susceptible pneumococci in adults: a case-control study. Scandinavian Journal of Infectious Disease 30(3):253–256
4. Pallares R, Linares J, Vadillo M, Cabellos C, Manresa F, Viladrich PF, Martin R, Gudiol F (1995) Resistance to penicillin and cephalosporin and mortality from severe pneumococcal pneumonia in Barcelona, Spain. New England Journal of Medicine 333(8):474–480
5. U.S.Congress, Office of Technology Assessment. Impacts of Antibiotic Resistant Bacteria. OTA-H-629 (Washington D.C. U.S. Government Printing Office, September 1995)
6. Dixon RE (1985) Economic costs of respiratory tract infections in the United States. American Journal of Medicine Vol 45
7. National Center for Health Statistics (1992) National Hospital Discharge Survey: Annual summary 1990. Vital Health Stat 13:1–225

Part 1
Antimicrobial Chemotherapy

CHAPTER 2

Antimicrobial Chemotherapy – Today

2

JOHN DAVID WILLIAMS

Abstract. Research on chemotherapy of infection and immunotherapy of infection started almost as soon as infection was found to be a cause of disease. Valuable agents came from dye stuffs and heavy metals; enhancement of immunity and vaccination were in use very quickly; antibiotics came later and added their own impact on treatment. As this century ends we are very rich in remedies and rich in problems surrounding them. We are still faced with many infections unresolved by treatment – new pathogens have emerged, resistance to therapy has increased and new complex therapy appears. Some areas where we may be in error today are:

- promoting resistance to therapy by inappropriate management
- blaming the wrong persons for causing the problems
- expecting genetics to solve the epidemiological problem and
- expecting guidelines drawn up by committees to provide ideal therapy for individual patients.

These subjects are presented as a brief survey of the agenda of the meeting.

Introduction

Antimicrobial treatment today consists of three elements: antibiotics, chemotherapy and immunotherapy. The aim of immunotherapy is to help the body's defences deal with the infectious organism. This area has produced enormous advances through active immunisation and it holds much promise for the future. Nevertheless, the two main planks on which we base current antimicrobial therapy remain chemotherapy and antibiotics. Chemotherapy can be described as chemistry versus biology. It uses chemical agents against the infectious microbes. Antibiotic therapy, on the other hand, uses the agents produced by microbes themselves against other microbes.

Historical Perspective

Chemotherapy arose in the last century out of the German dye industry. From these early dyes sprang 3 different 'lines': the red, the blue and the brightly coloured yellow. The red dye, prontosil rubrum, showed distinct antimicrobial activity and when hydrolysed, it gave rise to sulphanilamide and a wide range of subsequent sulphonamides. These were very useful chemotherapeutic agents in the middle part of this century.

The blue line is based on methylene blue. Methylene blue was used in the 1890's for malaria and for treatment of urinary tract infection. In more modern times, methylene blue was used to produce neuroleptic drugs, such as phenothiazines and the antihistamine drugs. Today, there is renewed interest in phenothiazines, especially with regard to their anti-mycobacterial activity, and in blood transfusion circles for their effects against viruses such as HIV and those causing hepatitis.

The yellow line is the most relevant for this symposium. This line was based on the yellow dye, amine acridine, and it's derivative mepacrine. One could easily pick out malaria patients because they were yellow from taking mepacrine. The first quinolone, nalidixic acid, is from the yellow line and the fluoroquinolones followed some time later. Moxifloxacin is the latest in the line of fluoroquinolone antibiotics.

Chemotherapy differs from antibiotic therapy. Chemotherapeutic agents attack the very fundamental building blocks of life. These are the essential agonists of all life processes, the DNA, the thymidylate pathway, and the universal energy source of man and microbes, ATP (adenosine triphosphate). Antibiotics have got much more specific targets; they are bigger molecules and have targets such as bacterial cell wall components and ribosomal elements.

The chemotherapeutic and antibiotic drugs we use today are derived from quite different sources, but have both undergone the same sorts of chemical manipulation and molecular change. As a result, antibiotics can be classified into 'lines' just like the chemotherapeutic agents. For example, there are three types of beta-lactam antibiotics, the penicillins (1940), cephalosporins (1960), and carbapenems (1980), with twenty years between the usage of each class.

The crossroads for beta-lactam compounds occurred in 1960 when ampicillin and cephalexin were produced. Ampicillin has enjoyed wide use, as have its various derivatives such as Bayer's mezlocillin and azlocillin. Cephalexin is now used primarily to treat urinary tract infections, especially during pregnancy. Nevertheless, cephalexin has been the role model for all subsequent cephalosporins because of its high bioavailability and its stability to beta-lactamases.

The key to beta-lactam antibiotics is their characteristic side-chains. Addition of an alpha-amino benzyl substituent on a penicillin produces ampicillin. The presence of the same side-chain on a cephalosporin nucleus produces cephalexin. Table 1 lists some examples of congruent side chain substituents in penicillins and cephalosporins. This illustrates the close relationship between all beta-lactams and explains their mirrored activity. Similar processes of chemical modification have been used in all other classes of antibiotics.

Table 1. Some examples of congruent side-chain substituents in penicillins and cephalosporins

Side chain	Penicillins	Cephalosporins
α-amino benzyl	(6) Ampicillin	(7) Cephalexin
dioxopiperazine	(6) Piperacillin	(7) Cefperazone
α-methoxy	(6) Temocillin	(7) Cefoxitin
oximino-amino-thiazole	(4) Aztreonam	(7) Ceftazidime

Driving forces for new antibiotic therapy

Resistance drives the search for new antimicrobial agents. This resistance is natural or acquired. Some organisms have strong natural defences against antimicrobials (such as the pseudomonads and enterococci) and others (such as Gram-negative rods and staphylococci) readily acquire antibiotic resistance.

New antimicrobials are also needed to satisfy the demand for convenience. People used to be quite happy to be cured. Today, they want high efficacy with no side effects and expect an oral formulation with infrequent dosing. As a result, drugs with high bioavailability and optimal pharmacokinetics are highly desired.

A word about guidelines

A third factor influencing antimicrobial therapy today is the growth of treatment guidelines. Guidelines have become extremely popular with individuals and especially with health maintenance organisations. What began with simple guidelines for endocarditis has spread to guidelines for urinary tract, respiratory and paediatric infections, and the list is growing.

Ten years ago, the diagnosis of the aetiological agent of respiratory tract infection was very difficult, but treatment was easy when one knew what to treat. These days, diagnosis is not necessary, but the treatment is very complex. Many guidelines are used to decide on which antibiotic mixtures to use to cover all eventualities.

Respiratory tract infections are complicated with multiple aetiological agents that vary with age and underlying disease, precipitating causes, area of the world, socio-economic status, race, colour, sex and occupation. The disease presents in different ways and so the ideal treatment should be very specific to aetiological diagnosis.

Treatment guidelines are definitely needed in places where there are few competent medical staff, a limited definition of disease syndrome and a small number of available antibiotics. For example, the WHO guidelines for treatment of pneumonia in less than one year-old infants [1] is used in villages with no trained medical personnel. It is based on easily measured criteria such as fever, respiratory rate and cyanosis, and employs simple antibiotics, such as co-trimoxazole, or amoxicillin (for moderate disease) and chloramphenicol (for severe disease).

Such guidelines have saved many lives, but are they necessary in the developed world? After years of study, our physicians should be able to use their skills in common respiratory tract infection. It is hoped that proper medical education in microbiology and infectious disease will reduce the need for mandatory treatment guidelines.

Are we losing the war against microbes?

Early in the 19th century, Paul Ehrlich summarised his three requirements for treatment of infection: efficacy, convenience, and low toxicity. Ehrlich was searching for the '*therapia sterilans magna*', the one dose treatment that would cure everything; kill all the germs and totally destroy microbes; and have a low chemotherapeutic index (defined as the minimum curative dose over the minimum toxic dose). Ehrlich believed that all microorganisms could be controlled with chemotherapeutic agents in this manner. Writing in 1913 he stated:

"*Now... the danger of (infectious) disease is to a great extent circumscribed as far as epidemics are concerned... the efforts of chemotherapeutics are to fill up the gaps left in the ring. The ordinary bacterial diseases (streptococcus, staphylococcus, coli, typhoid, dysentery and above all tuberculosis) still require a hard struggle. Nevertheless I look forward with full confidence... without being set down as an optimist put forward the view that in the next five years we will have advances of the highest importance to report.*" [2]

Perhaps Paul Ehrlich was a bit hopeful. It turns out that five years was not sufficient to cure infectious disease. The problem lay in the fact that the biology of Man and Microbe are more clearly related than was envisaged. They both share the same purines, the same amino acids and similar target pathways. New organisms have arisen where old ones fell. People survive today who would not have survived 40 years ago. The ultra small neonate, the very old, the immuno-compromised or chronically invaded host, all would all have died in 1947. These highly susceptible patients present today's greatest challenges in the fight against microbial infection.

Hospitals have proven to be a large part of the problem related to antibiotic resistance. They are the sites where resistance develops and Table 2 lists the many organisms that now cause hospital infections. It appears that 60 years of chemotherapy and antibiotics has favoured the survival of the 'unfittest'. Antibiotics provide cover for advanced surgery and other interventions, and the WHO motto [3] 'Health for All by 2000', should probably read 'Antibiotics for All by 2000'.

Today, man, animals and plants, all require antibiotics. Some may wonder whether we have reached the "Gotterdammerung" (Armageddon) of antibiotics. This is probably not the case. We still pick the golden apples that Wagner described, but the Valhalla of selective toxicity may be beyond our reach. Man and Microbe are twinned, just as Siegmund and Sieglinde, and we will always have to balance the effect on one versus the effect on the other.

Table 2. Organisms responsible for hospital infections in 1998

S. aureus	MRSA
Enterococci	VRE
Enterobacteria	Multi-antibiotic-resistant Gram-negative rods
P. aeruginosa and other species Anaerobes	
Yeasts and fungi	
Organisms of low pathogenicity in wide variety and with high level of resistance to antibiotics	

Ehrlich's predictions may still come to pass. Five years was perhaps too optimistic, but it is not unrealistic to expect that the next 50 years will continue to bring many exciting advances in antimicrobial therapy.

References

1. The World Health Organization (1995) The Management of Acute Respiratory Tract Infections in Children: Practical guidelines for outpatient care
2. Ehrlich P (1913) Chemotherapeutics: scientific principles, methods and results. Lancet II: 445–451
3. World Health Organization, Health for All in the 21st Century Policy, adopted May 16, 1998

CHAPTER 3

Antimicrobial Chemotherapy – Tomorrow   3

HARTMUT LODE

Abstract. An increasing incidence of problems with bacterial resistance to antibiotics has emerged. Many different diseases are becoming more important, as a result of the ageing population. Resistant and newer pathogens have appeared and spread rapidly. These major threats to global health require new strategies for future chemotherapy for bacterial diseases. Optimal use of available drugs, identification of resistance mechanisms and rational development of new drugs are required. Drug development will target specific mechanisms involved in the pathogen's attack on cells. New antimicrobials in development will be reviewed. The future of infectious diseases and their control will be determined by many factors, including improved diagnosis, changing aetiology, more aggressive medical procedures, population characteristics, cost benefit of the proposed treatments and the political will to undertake them. Infectious disease in the future will be influenced by the increase in age, crowding and mobility of the population.

Perspectives of Infectious Diseases in the Beginning of the Next Century

In the next 10 to 20 years many changes are likely to influence disease emergence. Increases in urban crowding and the age of the population are both expected to have an impact on infectious disease, as are the rise in world travel, global warming and the growth of microbial drug resistance. In terms of the human race, elements to be considered include the extremes of age, poverty, malnutrition and population control. Individual factors such as sexual behaviour, smoking, personal hygiene, alcohol consumption, immune status and, again, frequent travel must also be included. For the microbe, the next century will hold changes in microbial genetics and in resistance. Commensals will become pathogens in specific patient populations, more pathogens will produce toxins, and 'new' organisms are likely to emerge.

Advances in diagnosis are expected to improve future antimicrobial therapy. New rapid microbiologic diagnostic kits may provide benefits, as might immunologic tools such as gene probes and radiologic tools such as magnetic radiation. Logic-oriented diagnostic systems may also have an impact on clinical work performed in both hospital and outpatient settings.

Medical practice after the year 2000 will involve a greater number of immunosuppressed patients. There will be more major surgery in the elderly. Transplantations and invasive procedures will be performed more frequently. The use of prostheses is expected to increase, as is 'over-the-counter' prescribing.

Cost will remain a big consideration, especially for the pharmaceutical industry which must invest around $ 500 million U.S in order to develop a new drug. The cost-benefit of any new antibiotic, it's commercial and political aspects, will be important future considerations, as will the ability of developing countries to purchase these new antibiotics.

Diseases likely to become more important in the new millennium include the measles, where the incidence is expected to rise as a result of today's poor compliance with immunisation. Many difficult diseases are also becoming more important due to population ageing. Hepatitis A virus mortality is 10 % in adults over 65 [1]; thus the different types of hepatitis (Hepatitis A, C, E, and now F), are likely to become more prevalent. Fortunately, Hepatitis B will be manageable with vaccination programs, but tuberculosis will continue to cause difficulties as a result of persistent drug and compliance problems. Pneumonia, where mortality is 50 % in adults over 65 years [2], will continue to be the leading infectious disease in industrial countries. While meningitis and encephalitis will still be important causes of disease, especially in the Third World.

Microbes that are expected to be problematic after the year 2000 include methicillin-resistant *Staphloccoccus aureus* (MRSA). Currently 20 % of bacteraemic patients have MRSA [3] and this is expected to rise. Another problem is penicillin-resistant pneumococcus. There is a 40 % incidence of this resistant strain in Spain [4], and it will soon spread to the rest of Europe. Other microbial pathogens that are likely to cause problems include penicillin-tolerant viridans streptococci (endocarditis organisms), multi-resistant *Klebsiella*, which produce extended spectrum beta-lactamases, *Pseudomonas aeruginosa, Stenotrophmonas maltophilia, Mycobacterium tuberculosis* and *Mycobacterium leprae* (especially in the Third World).

With regard to bacterial resistance, the problems with *Streptococcus pneumoniae* have already been mentioned. There is also the recent report of vancomycin-resistant *Staphylococcus aureus* [5]. Table 1 lists some more common resistant bacteria. In general, there appear to be a lot of problems in the Gram-positive field. The following statement from Bob Moellering [6] emphasises the point, *'in the past decade, (he) has seen a crescendo of problems with multidrug resistant Gram-positive bacteria including methicillin-resistant staphylococci, penicillin-resistant pneumococci and vancomycin-resistant enterococci. The latter are particular vexing because several strains of VRE are resistance to all available antibiotics'.*

Table 1
Some common drug-resistant bacteria

Drug	Resistant Bacteria
Penicillin	*S. pneumoniae*
Ampicillin	*E. faecium*
Vancomycin	*S. aureus*
Quinolones	*Salmonella/shigella* ssp.
Amphotericin	*Candida* ssp.
Metronidazole	*B. fragilis*
Cephalosporin	*Enterobacter* spp.
Isoniazid/rifampicin	*M. tuberculosis*

Focussing specifically on *Staphylococcus*, the future holds increasing resistance. MRSA will persist, as will the homeless, drug addicts and ageing/elderly cohorts. Resistance to fluoroquinolones is also growing and resistance of MRSA to ciprofloxacin will soon be >80% [7]. Isolates will become resistant to macrolides and aminoglycosides, and plasmids will develop resistance to vancomycin and teicoplanin.

In summary, new treatment strategies are needed for changing aetiologies, new pathogens, more resistant old pathogens, more elderly patients with severe underlying disease, more immuno-compromised patients and more infections in the hospitals due to aggressive diagnostic and therapeutic methods.

Some New Antibacterials Being Developed for the Next 5-10 Years

Paul Ehrlich, who worked in Berlin and Frankfurt early in this century, listed his four ingredients for success (The Four German G's) [8]. These are the elements required for the successful development of a new antibiotic.

Geld – money
Geduld – patience
Geschick – cleverness
Glück – luck

Several therapeutic classes are of interest for future antimicrobial development. There is a search for better beta-lactams, penems, macrolides, ketolides, everninomycins, fluoroquinolones, streptogramins, oxazolidinones, and glycopeptides. In this meeting, the new fluoroquinolones such as gatifloxacin, gemifloxacin, grepafloxacin, trovafloxacin and of course, moxifloxacin, are especially relevant.

Table 2 lists some fluoroquinolones currently under development in Asia [9]. Note that Toyama's T3811 was designed without the fluorine in position 6 in order to reduce phototoxicity (Fig. 1). Of the oxazolidinones listed in Table 3 [10], Bayer is developing thienyloxazolidinone and pyridyloxazolidinone, and perhaps in 3 to 5 years they will be holding another meeting to discuss these new agents. Schering's everninomycin [11] (Fig. 2) is a very large molecule and its

Table 2. Fluoroquinolone compounds under development

Chemical Family	Antibacterial spectrum	Code no./name	Pharmaceutical company
Fluoroquinolones	GP, GN, I	T-3811	Toyama (Toyama, Japan)
	GP, GN, I	WQ 3034/WQ 2724	Wakunaga Pharm. (Hiroshima, Japan)
	GP, GN, I	KRQ 10.018	Korea Res. Inst. Chem. Technol. (Taejon, Korea)

GP, Gram-positive; *GN*, Gram-negative; *I*, intracellular bacteria.

Fig. 1
The molecular structure of
toyama T-3811

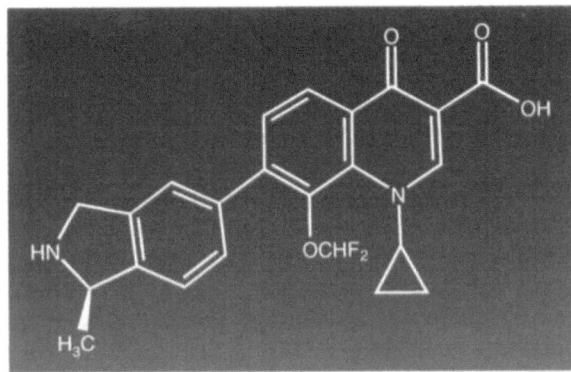

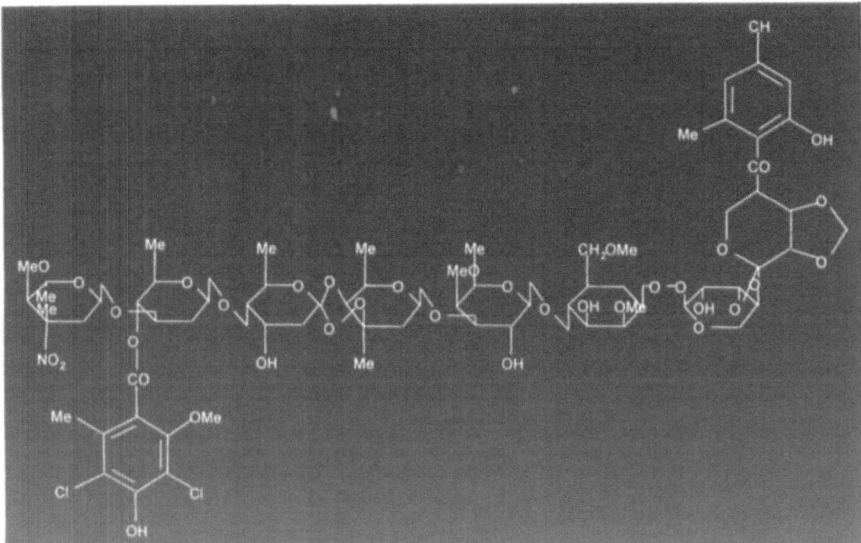

Fig. 2. The molecular structure of everninomycin

Table 3. Oxazolidinone compounds under development

Chemical Family	Antibacterial spectrum	Code no./name	Pharmaceutical company
Oxazolidinones	GP	PNU 101.099	Pharmacia Upjohn (Kalamzoo, MI)
	GP	PNU 101.850	Pharmacia Upjohn
Thienyloxazolidinones	GP		Bayer AG (Lerverkusen, Germany)
Pyridyloxazolidinones	GP		Bayer AG

GP, Gram-positive.

mode of action has not yet been fully elucidated. However, it will be interesting to observe this agent's performance in clinical trials.

Considerations for Future Drug Development

There are several stages in the bacterial cycle of infection, which are available for potential drug intervention. New drugs could be developed to prevent the surface protein interaction between pathogen and cell. The entry of pathogens into the cells could be blocked, as could pathogen replication. Another strategy would be to inhibit the growth and development of pathogens by targeting the critical pathogen-specific enzymes.

Much has been learned regarding viral infection (e. g. HIV) and this should be useful in similar situations with bacterial infections. Potential therapeutic interventions include blocking the transfer of pathogen macromolecule between specific intracellular compartments. Critical steps in the maturation of pathogens could also be blocked, as could the interaction with host factors essential for pathogen reactivation, replication and persistence. Finally, another area that is available for future development, is the identification and exploitation of bacterial virulence factors in order to target delivery of drugs to desired sites.

Conclusion

In conclusion, antimicrobial therapy "tomorrow" must involve more appropriate use of available antimicrobial drugs. There must be better identification of resistance mechanisms and more rational development of new drugs. Innovative approaches such as adherence inhibition and immune modulation should be used as a basis for future antimicrobial development.

References – Selected readings

Forbes A, Williams R (1990) Changing epidemiology and clinical aspects of hepatitis A. Br Me Bull 46:303–306

Kollett MH, Silver P, Murphy DM, Trovillion E (1995) The effect of late-onset ventilator-associated pneumonia in determining patient mortality. Chest 108:1655–1662

Vincent JI, Bihari DJ, Suter PM, Bruining HA, White J, Nicolas-Chanoin MH (1995) The prevalence of nosocomial infection in intensive care units in Europe. JAMA 274:639–644

Ewig S, Ruiz M, Torres A, Marco F, Martinez JA, Sanchez M, Mensa J (1999) Pneumonia acquired in the community through drug-resistant Streptococcus pneumoniae. Am J Respir Crit Care 159:1835–1842

Pallares R, Linares J, Vadillo M, Cabellos C, Manresa F, Viladrich F, Martin R, Gudiol F (1995) Resistance to penicillin and cephalosporin and mortality from severe pneumococcal pneumonia in Barcelona, Spain. N Engl J Med 333:474–480

Hiramatsu K, Hanaki H, Ino T, Yabuta K, Oguri T, Tenover FC (1997) Methicillin-resistant Staphylococus aureus clinical strain with reduced vancomycin susceptibility. J Antimicrob Chemother 40:135–136

Smith TL, Pearson ML, Wilcox KR et al. (1999) Emergence of vancomycin resistance in Staphylococcus aureus. N Engl J Med 340:493–501

Sieradzki K, Roberts RB, Haber SW, Tomasz A (1999) The development of vancomycin resistance in a patient with methicillin-resistant Staphylococcus aureus infection. N Engl J Med 340:517–523

Moellering RC Jr (1999) A novel antimicrobial agent joins the battle against resistant bacteria (editorial). Annals of Internal Medicine 130(2):155–157

Moellering RC (1998) Problems with antimicrobial resistance in gram-positive cocci. Clin Infect Dis 26:1177–1178

Israeli A (1998) Paul Ehrlich's ingredients for success (letter). The Lancet 352(9141):1712

Bryskier A (1998) Novelties in the field of anti-infectives in 1997. Clin Infect Dis 27:865–883

Hayashi K, Todo Y, Hamamoto S et al. (1997) T-3811, a novel des -F(6)-quinolone: synthesis and in vitro activity of 7-(isoindolin-5-yl) derivates (abstract F-158). In: Program and abstracts of the 37th Interscience Conference on Antimicrobial Agents and Chemotherapy. Washington, DC. American Society for Microbiology, 173

Takahata M, Misuyama F, Yamashiro Y et al. (1997) T-3811, a novel des-F(6)-quinolone: study of pharmacokinetics in animals (abstract F-160). In: Program and abstracts of the 37th Interscience Conference on Antimicrobiall Agents and Chemotherapy. Washington, DC. American Society for Microbiology, 173

Amano H, Hayashi N, Oshita Y, Nino Y, Yazaki A (1997) WQ 2724 and WQ 2743 novel fluoroquinolones: In vitro and in vivo activities, pharmacokinetics and toxicity (abstract F-163). In: Program and abstracts of the 37th Interscience Conference on Antimicrobial Agents and Chemotherapy. Washington, DC. American Society for Microbiology, 174

Oshita Y, Yazaki A (1997) In vitro studies with WQ-3034, a newly synthesized acidic fluoroquinolone (abstract F-164). In: Program and abstracts of the 37th Interscience Conference on Antimicrobial Agents and Chemotherapy. Washington DC. American Society for Microbiology, 174

Bryskier A (1998) Novelties in the field of anti-infectives in 1997. Clin Infect Dis 27:865–883

Gadwood RC, Kamdar BV, Sims SM, Martin IJ, Zurenko GE, Ford CW (1997) Synthesis of oxazolidinone antibacterial agents incorporating morpholine and piperazine N-oxides: oxazolidinone prodrugs having high water solubility (abstract F-20). In: Program and abstracts of the 37th Interscience Conference on Antimicrobial Agents and Chemotherapy. Washington, DC. American Society for Microbiology, 149

Ulanowicz DA, Brickner SJ, Ford CW, Zurenko GE (1997) Synthesis and biological activity of N-acetyl modified analogs of oxazolidinone antibacterial agents linezolid and eperezolid (abstract F-21). In: Program and abstracts of the 37th Interscience Conference on Antimicrobial Agents and Chemotherapy. Washington, DC: American Society for Microbiology, 149

Bartel S, Endermann R, Guarnieri W et al. (1997) Synthesis and antibacterial activity of novel hereroaryl oxazolidinones I: Thiophenyl oxazolidinones (abstract F-17). In: Program and abstracts of the 37th Interscience Conference on Antimicrobial Agents and Chemotherapy. Washington, DC: American Society for Microbiology, 149

Bartel S, Endermann R, Guarnieri W et al. (1997) Synthesis and antibacterial activity of novel heteroxyl oxazolidinones II: Pyridyl oxazolidinones (abstract F-18). In: Program and abstracts of the 37th Interscience Conference on Antimicrobial Agents and Chemotherapy. Washington, DC. American Society for Microbiology, 149

Bartel S, Endermann R, Guarnieri W et al. (1997) Synthesis and antibacterial activity of novel heteroxyl oxazolidinones III: activities against clinically important gram-positive cocci (abstract F-19). In: Program and abstracts of the 37th Interscience Conference on Antimicrobial Agents and Chemotherapy. Washington, DC American Society for Microbiology, 149

Vesga O, Craig WA (1997) In vivo pharmacodynamic activity of SCH 27,8995SCH (Ziracin) and everninomicin antibiotic (abstract A-32). In: Program and abstracts of the 37th Interscience Conference on Antimicrobial Agents and Chemotherapy. Washington, DC. American Society for Microbiology, 6

Banfield CR, Glue P, Affrime M. et al. (1997) Multiple-dose safety, tolerance and pharma-cokinetics of Ziracin (SCH 27,899): a new, novel oligosaccharide antibiotic (abstract A-114). In: Program and abstracts of the 37th Interscience Conference on Antimicrobial Agents and Chemotherapy. Washington, DC. American Society for Microbiology, 6

Menon S, Pai S, Banfield CR, Cayen M, Affrime MB, Batra V (1997) Effect of gender on the pharmacokinetics of Ziracin (SCH 27,899) in healthy volunteers (abstract A-113). In: Program and abstracts of the 37th Interscience Conference on Antimicrobial Agents and Chemotherapy. Washington, DC. American Society for Microbiology, 23

Part 2
Pre-clinical

CHAPTER 4

Pre-clinical Microbiology – Streptococcus Pneumoniae

4

REGINE HAKENBECK

Abstract. *Streptococcus pneumoniae* is rapidly becoming resistant to beta-lactam antibiotics. An increasing association of penicillin resistance with that against macrolides is documented. Multiple antibiotic resistance phenotypes are also common. This phenomenon requires the development of new effective antimicrobials. Moxifloxacin is a highly effective new fluoro-quinolone. It is 2–4 times more active than sparfloxacin and ciprofloxacin, and is similar in activity to trovafloxacin. It is active against pneumococci regardless of the resistance profile of the strains. In *S. pneumoniae* resistant to fluoroquinolones, mutations occur first in the ParC subunit of topoisomerase IV followed by secondary mutations in the GyrA subunit of DNA gyrase. Efflux-related resistance mechanisms have also been reported. High level resistance requires multiple alterations in the target proteins.

Introduction

Pneumococcus is still one of the major pathogens in the world. It causes pneu-monia, sinusitis, acute otitis and meningitis, diseases that are very often com-plicated by additional side effects. It is also a minor bacterial pathogen in bronchitis. Pneumococcal infections are usually treated with beta-lactams, but a 1977 hospital outbreak in South Africa revealed some alarming trends [1, 2]. Isolated strains of *Streptococcus pneumoniae* were found to be resistant to beta-lactams, penicillin as well as cephalosporins, erythromycin, chloramphenicol, clindamycin, tetracycline, trimethoprim sulphate, streptomycin, rifampin, and gentamicin. The resistant organisms were only susceptible to vancomycin, bacitracin and novobiocin, none of which were used initially during the out-break.

It is disturbing to note that, not only did the strains develop multiple-drug resistance, but also their resistance levels against beta-lactams increased. In 1940 pneumococci were generally susceptible to beta-lactams with a minimum inhi-bitory concentration (MIC) of about 0.01 µg/mL. Meanwhile, isolates with MIC values rising from 0.6 up to 4 µg/mL beta-lactam have been reported. In Europe, Spain and Hungary remain 'hot-spots' for beta-lactam and multiple antibiotic resistant pneumococci where about 50% of isolates have MIC values greater than 1 µg/mL [3, 4].

The observed decrease in antibiotic activity is significant, especially since one begins to realise that the pathogen may not necessarily be the driving force be-hind the development of resistance. Resistance may have evolved in commensal streptococci, subsequently spreading into the pneumococcal population via gene transfer [5]. Thus, in order to understand resistance, investigations of the pathogen alone are not sufficient. Organisms that contribute to the genepool which is available for the pathogen also have to be considered. A striking example is a *Streptococcus mitis* isolate from Germany with MIC values for beta-lactams above 60 µg/mL which was transferable to a laboratory strain of *S. pneumoniae* without affecting growth parameters of the transformant [6].

Results and Discussion

Given the rise in resistance, it is important to determine whether we have the antibiotics necessary to treat pneumococcal infections. An in-vitro study compared the activity of several antibiotics against three populations of *S. pneumoniae* (Table 1). Data showed that moxifloxacin had a good MIC_{90} distribution. Values for penicillin-sensitive, penicillin-intermediate and penicillin-resistant types ranged from 0.06 to 0.25 µg/mL. Therefore, moxifloxacin can be used for the whole population of drug-resistant pneumococci. It is also of note that none of the other fluoroquinolones tested showed comparably low MIC_{90} values [7].

Figure 1 plots MIC values against the number of pneumococci strains with that minimum inhibitory concentration. There were over a thousand strains tested, most of which were penicillin-sensitive, with only 30 strains that were penicillin-resistant (note the small peak around 2 µg/mL). Moxifloxacin and trovafloxacin MIC values showed equal distribution, with maximum values at about 0.12 µg/mL. Ciprofloxacin and levofloxacin shared similar MIC profiles, with peak values occurring at 1 µg/mL. MIC distributions for ofloxacin and lomefloxacin peaked at 2 and 4 µg/mL, respectively. The lomefloxacin peak, however, had a prominent shoulder shifted towards the higher MIC values. Based on these data, moxifloxacin and trovafloxacin showed the best activity profiles [8].

When comparing the activity of quinolone-resistant pneumococci against moxifloxacin, sparfloxacin and ciprofloxacin, moxifloxacin again had the highest

Table 1. The activity of antibiotics against three different populations of *S. pneumoniae*. Penicillin susceptibilities: sensitive (Pen S), intermediate (Pen I), resistant (Pen R)

	Activity MIC_{90} (µg/mL)		
	Pen S	Pen I	Pen R
Amoxicillin	0.03–0.06	1–2	8
Cefuroxime	0.06–0.25	2–4	8–16
Clarithromycin	0.03–0.25	4–64	32–>256
TMP/SMX	1	8–16	8–16
Levofloxacin	1–2	1–2	1–2
Grepafloxacin	0.25–0.5	0.25–0.5	0.25–0.5
Gatifloxacin	0.5	0.5	0.5
Moxifloxacin	0.06–0.25	0.12–0.25	0.12–0.25

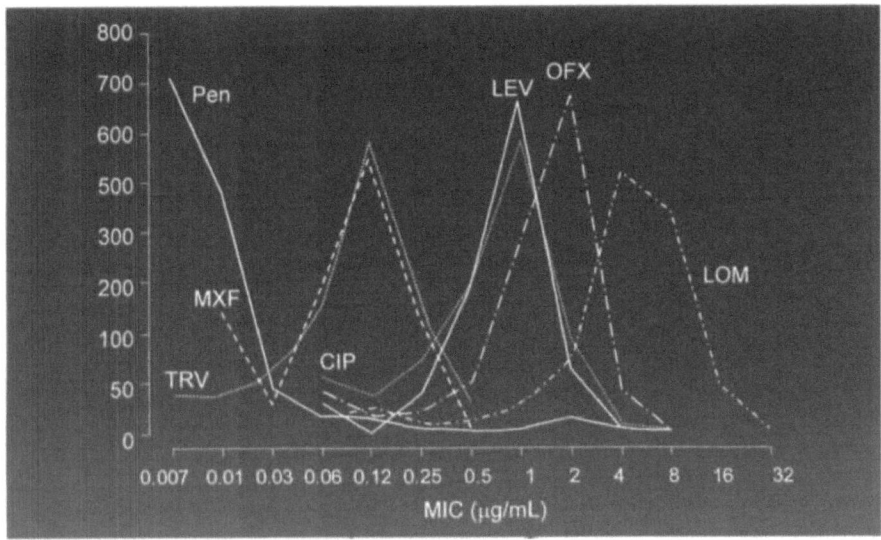

Fig. 1. The impact of penicillin resistance on quinolone susceptibilities. TRV – trovafloxacin, MXF – moxifloxacin, Pen – penicillin, CIP – ciprofloxacin, LEV – levofloxacin, OFX – ofloxacin, LOM – lomefloxacin

activity against the resistant organisms [9]. The results suggested, however, that high level resistance to quinolones was associated with high level resistance to beta-lactams. A new study comparing the efficacy of different antibiotics using around 2,000 beta-lactam resistant strains would allow for proper statistical evaluation of this association.

Moving from in-vitro to in-vivo efficacy, Fig. 2 illustrates the effect of moxifloxacin against *Staphylococcus aureus* and *S. pneumoniae* in the rat. The animals were administered 100 mg/kg moxifloxacin either 1 h or 24 h after infection with the pathogen. Moxifloxacin provided rapid eradication of the pneumococcus bacteria in those rats treated 1 h post-infection. This eradication was significantly slower when treatment was delayed. The same held true for *Staphylococcus*, which showed a rapid decline after early moxifloxacin administration, and a slower drop 23 h later [10].

A comparison of the activity of selected antibiotics against Gram-positive bacteria (see Table 2), again showed that moxifloxacin was in the top range in terms of efficacy. This was true for MIC_{50} and MIC_{90} values as well as for whole range values [11].

With regard to resistance, there are two mechanisms that may result in its development against fluoroquinolones. The first is a nonspecific efflux mechanism in the genes that are mediating that mechanism for Gram-negative and Gram-positive bacteria. The second mechanism involves the specific fluoroquinolone targets. These are the two topoisomerases of class II, gyrase consisting of the two subunits encoded by *gyrA* and *gyrB*, and topoisomerase IV (*parC* and *parE*). Both the GyrA and the ParC subunit contain the so-called QRDR domain (quinolone resistance-determining region) which interacts with the

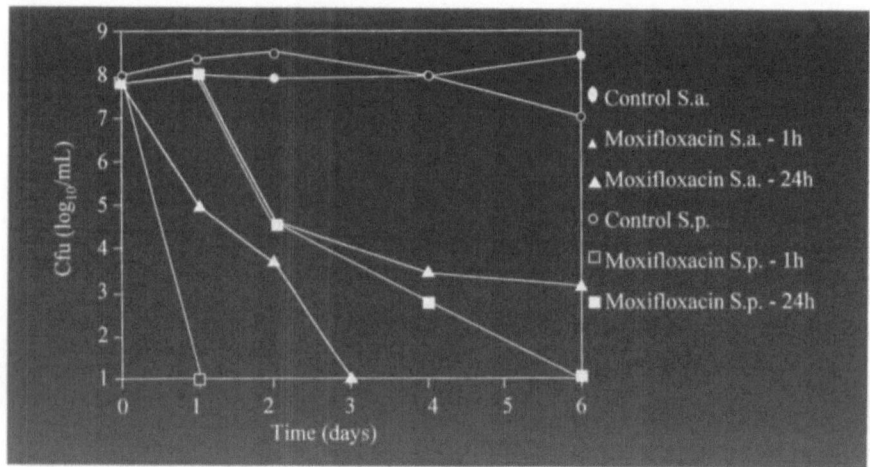

Fig. 2. The in-vivo efficacy of moxifloxacin against *S. aureus* (S.a.) and *S. pneumoniae* (S.p.) in the rat after administration 1 h and 24 h post-infection

Table 2. The activity of fluoroquinolones and other antibiotics against Gram-positive bacteria

Bacteria (n)	Drug	Activity, MICs (µg/mL)		
		50%	90%	Range
streptococci (10) Group A	Moxifloxacin	0.125	0.5	0.062–0.5
	Trovafloxacin	0.125	0.5	0.031–0.5
	Ciprofloxacin	⊢————————————⊣		0.06–2
	Ampicillin	0.015	0.031	0.007–0.031
	Nafcillin	0.015	0.015	0.003–0.015
	Vancomycin	0.25	0.25	0.25
streptococci (10) Group B	Moxifloxacin	0.25	0.25	0.062–0.25
	Trovafloxacin	0.125	0.125	0.125
	Ciprofloxacin	0.5	1	0.5–1
	Ampicillin	0.25	0.25	0.25
	Nafcillin	0.25	0.25	0.25
	Vancomycin	0.5	0.5	0.5
S. pneumoniae	Moxifloxacin	0.125	0.25	0.125–0.25
	Trovafloxacin	0.125	0.125	0.015–0.125
	Ampicillin	0.25	2	0.031–16
	Nafcillin	2	8	0.031–16
	Vancomycin	0.25	0.25	0.25

Table 3
The activity of moxifloxacin, sparfloxacin and cipro-floxacin against laboratory-created quinolone-resistant strains of S. pneumoniae

Organism	Activity MIC (µg/mL)		
	Moxi	Spar	Cipro
SPn 5907	0.06	0.25	2
SPn 5929*	0.06	0.5	8
R6tr 5929*	0.06	0.25	16
R6p16b 1b4+	16	64	256

* No mutation in gyr/par.
+ Mutation at gyrA(2)/parC(2).

DNA substrate. Most mutations that confer resistance are located within this domain.

In E. coli and other Gram-negative bacteria, the gyrase is the primary target for resistance. In Gram-positive bacteria such as S. aureus and S. pneumoniae, however, the topoisomerase IV enzyme is a primary target and mutations in the gyrase are responsible for higher resistance levels.

The ATPase domain of the gyrase is structurally related to the conserved domain of histidine protein kinases of bacterial two-component signal trans-ducing systems. Thus, topoisomerases contain domains, besides the regions that are targeted by quinolones, that may provide targets for other, as yet undis-covered, antimicrobial compounds.

The relationship between quinolone resistance and moxifloxacin activity was investigated using laboratory-created resistant strains of S. pneumoniae [12] (see Table 3). The sensitive strain SPn 5907 was used as a control and ciprofloxacin (4 µg/mL) was used as the selective agent. The selected strains (Spn 5929) were more or less exclusively resistant to ciprofloxacin. There was a slight increase in the sparfloxacin MIC value (0.25 to 0.5 µg/mL), but no corresponding change in the moxifloxacin MIC value (0.06 µg/mL). This resistance was apparently related to a target independent efflux mechanism (no mutation in gyrA or parC).

Using a ciprofloxacin resistant transformant obtained with SPn 5907 DNA, the mutant R6p 16b 1b4 was obtained after stepwise selection with pefloxacin (16 µg/mL) and Bay y3118 (Bay y3118; 1 µg/mL followed by 4 µg/mL selective concentration), resulting in MIC values of 256 µg/mL for ciprofloxacin and 16 µg/mL for moxifloxacin. This documents the resistance potential obtainable in only a few selection steps and again, the better activity of moxifloxacin com-pared to other quinolones especially ciprofloxacin.

Conclusion

Moxifloxacin shows good in-vitro activity against S. pneumoniae; this includes penicillin-sensitive, intermediate and resistant strains as well as quinolone-resistant pneumococci. Its efficacy has been proven in animal models for both S. pneumoniae and S. aureus, and laboratory-selection experiments reveal that moxifloxacin has a low propensity for the development of drug resistance in pneumococci.

References

1. Feldman C, Kallenbach JM, Miller SD, Thorburn JR, Koornhof HJ (1985) Community – acquired pneumonia due to penicillin – resistant pneumococci. New England Journal of Medicine 313:615–617
2. Jacobs MR, Koornhof HJ, Robins-Browne RM, Stevenson CM, Vermak ZA, Freiman I et al. (1978) Emergence of multiple resistant pneumococci. New England Journal of Medicine 299:735–740
3. Baquero F (1995) Pneumococcal resistance to beta-lactam antibiotics: a global geographic overview. Microbial Drug Resistance 1(2):115–120. Review
4. Schutze GE, Kaplan SL, Jacobs RF (1994) Resistant pneumococcus: a worldwide problem. Infection 22(4):233–237
5. Hakenbeck R (1999) beta-Lactam-Resistant Streptococcus pneumoniae: Epidemiology and Evolutionary Mechanism. Chemotherapy 45(2):83–94
6. Hakenbeck R, Konig A, Kern I, van der Linden M, Keck W, Billot-Klein D et al. (1998) Acquisition of five high-Mr penicillin-binding protein variants during transfer of high-level beta-lactam resistance from Streptococcus mitis to Streptococcus pneumoniae. Journal of Bacteriology 180(7):1831–1840
7. Blondeau JM, Yaschuk Y, Suter M, Vaughan D (1999) In-vitro susceptibility of 1982 respiratory tract pathogens and 1921 urinary tract pathogens against 19 antimicrobial agents: a Canadian multicentre study. Canadian Multicentre Study Group. Journal of Antimicrobial Chemotherapy 43(A):3–23
8. Buxbaum A, Straschil U, Moser C, Graninger W, Georgopoulos A (1999) Comparative susceptibility to penicilin and quinolones of 1385 streptococcus pneumoniae esolatis. Austrian Bacterial Surveillance Network. Journal of Antimicrobial Chemotherapy 43 Suppl. B:13–18
9. Brueggemann AB, Kugler KC, Doern GV (1997) In vitro activity of BAY 12-8039, a novel 8-methoxyquinolone, compared to activities of six fluoroquinolones against Streptococcus pneumoniae, Haemophilus influenzae, and Moraxella cattarrhalis. Antimicrobial Agents and Chemotherapy 41(7):1594–1597
10. Dalhoff A (1998) In Programme and Abstracts of the Eight International Conference on Infectious Diseases, Boston, MA
11. Malathum K, Singh KV, Murray BE (1998) In vitro activity of moxifloxacin against Gram-positive bacteria. In International Congress of Antimicrobial Agents and Chemotherapy, Abstract E204
12. Zeller V, Janoir C, Kitzis MD, Gutmann L, Moreau NJ (1997) Active efflux as a mechanism of resistance to ciprofloxacin in Streptococcus pneumoniae. Antimicrobial Agents and Chemotherapy 41(9):1973–1978

CHAPTER 5

Pre-clinical Microbiology – Gram-positive Cocci   5

SILVANO ESPOSITO

Abstract. Despite increased funding of health care and medical research in the field of bacterial infections, the secular trend of morbidity and mortality caused by bacterial infections has likely increased due to emerging pathogens and to bacterial resistance. Gram-positive cocci play an important role in the aetiology of bacterial infections in both hospital and community settings. A special CDC Committee (Atlanta, GA, USA) recently identified five major priorities to fight antibiotic resistance: *Enterococcus* spp., *Staphylococcus* spp., *Mycobacterium tuberculosis*, *Streptococcus pneumoniae* and *Neisseria gonorrhoeae*. Three priorities concern Gram-positive cocci, therefore agents active against these organisms are welcome. Moxifloxacin has greater antibacterial activity against *E. faecalis* and *E. faecium* than ampicillin and ciprofloxacin. It is also active against some strains of vancomycin-resistant enterococci, against MSSA and, in contrast to previous generations of fluoroquinolones, against MRSA. These data suggest that moxifloxacin represents an attractive option for difficult-to-treat infections. Although *Streptococcus pyogenes* is not a priority identified by the CDC, it is of concern due to the development of resistance to macrolides. Moxifloxacin has excellent antibacterial activity against GABHS, which is not affected by macrolide resistance. Its use may be indicated for treatment of *S. pyogenes*-related diseases in adults with a history of allergy to beta-lactams.

The purpose of this chapter is to review recent trends in Gram-positive infections and to investigate moxifloxacin's potential in the treatment of these diseases.

Despite increased spending on health care and research, the incidence of bacterial disease and resistance is increasing, as is related mortality. Money alone does not appear to show results, and this is illustrated by the trend in pneumonia-related deaths (Fig. 1). Mortality due to pneumonia declined rapidly early in this century, then around the 1950's it reached a steady-state level. Despite the introduction of new antibiotics, the pneumonia mortality rate has not dropped significantly since then. In fact, recent data show a slight increase [1].

The increased mortality is probably due to changes in the pathogens themselves. For instance, the aetiology of serious infectious diseases, such as nosocomial-acquired sepsis, is moving from Gram-negative to Gram-positive bacteria [2]. In 1981–1983, Gram-positive cocci were responsible for 42% of nosocomial-acquired sepsis, but by the end of the decade this had risen to 55%. At the same time there was a decrease in sepsis due to Gram-negative rods, from 52% of cases in 1981–1983 to 29% in 1991–1992.

Given these changes, the US Center for Disease Control set priorities in their programmes to fight antibiotic resistance [3]. Of the five bacteria that have been identified; *Streptococcus pneumoniae*, *Neisseria gonorrhoeae*, *Mycobacterium*

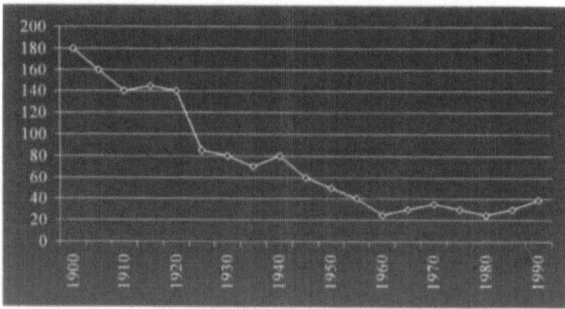

Fig. 1
Mortality rate for pneumonia
from 1900 to 1990.
N per 100,000 persons

tuberculosis, Staphylococcus spp. and *Enterococcus* spp., three of them are Gram-positive bacteria.

The incidence of vancomycin-resistant enterococci (VRE) [4] in the US illustrates the trend toward increasing resistance in Gram-positive bacteria. In 1989, VRE was almost unknown, yet only five years later, the incidence had reached 14% and recently, it has risen even more. Methicillin-resistant staphylococci (MRS) [5] emerged over a much longer period of time, perhaps 20 to 25 years. In 1975, the incidence of this resistance was almost negligible, in 1991 it had reached 35% and today it is even more prevalent. Given these figures, it is obvious that any antibiotic with activity against Gram-positive bacteria is welcome.

The in-vitro susceptibility of *Enterococcus faecalis* to selected antibiotics was compared using 43 strains, some vancomycin-sensitive and some vancomycin-resistant. Results are tabulated in Table 1. The MIC_{50} value for moxifloxacin was 0.5 μg/mL, while that for ciprofloxacin, ampicillin and vancomycin was 1 μg/mL [6]. Thus, at 0.5 μg/mL *Enterococcus faecalis* was susceptible to moxifloxacin in at least 50% of cases. Similar data by Woodcock et al. [7], using 20 strains of *E. faecium* showed that moxifloxacin was as active as ciprofloxacin, but less active than trovafloxacin.

In terms of MRSA (methicillin-resistant *Staphylococcus aureus*), moxifloxacin had much better activity than ciprofloxacin, but comparable activity to trovafloxacin, teicoplanin and vancomycin [8] (Table 2).

Streptococcus pyogenes is not considered to be a top priority in the fight against infectious disease. However, in the United States, there are 40 million

Table 1
The in-vitro activity of moxifloxacin and selected antibiotics against *Enterococcus faecalis* (43 strains)

Antibiotic	MIC_{50}	MIC_{90}	Range
	μg/mL	μg/mL	μg/mL
Moxifloxacin	0.5	8	0.25–32
Trovafloxacin	0.5	16	0.125–64
Ciprofloxacin	1	32	0.5–128
Ampicillin	1	4	1–16
Nafcillin	8	32	4–>256
Vancomycin	1	2	1–>256

Table 2
The in-vitro activity of
moxifloxacin and selected
antibiotics against MRSA
(60 strains)

Antibiotic	MIC$_{50}$	MIC$_{90}$	Range
	µg/mL	µg/mL	µg/mL
Moxifloxacin	1	2	≤0.03–8
Trovafloxacin	0.5	4	≤0.03–8
Ciprofloxacin	16	64	≤0.03–128
Quinupristin/ dalfopristin	1	1	≤0.03–2
Teicoplanin	1	2	≤0.03–4
Vancomycin	1	1	≤0.03–2

Table 3
The in-vitro activity of fluoroquinolones against erythromycin-resistant *Streptococcus
pyogenes*

Antibiotic	MIC90	Range
	µg/mL	µg/mL
Moxifloxacin	0.12	0.06–0.25
Ciprofloxacin	2	0.12–2
Ofloxacin	4	0.5–4
Sparfloxacin	0.5	0.12–2

cases of pharyngo-tonsillitis caused by *S. pyogenes* per year. Pharyngo-tonsillitis represents the third most common disease in the United States, and these data should be kept in mind given the re-emergence of serious pyogenes-related infections [9].

The development of macrolide resistance in *S. pyogenes* is also disturbing. In Italy, there are approximately 10 million cases of pharyngo-tonsillitis each year. Data from Naples showed that between 1993 and 1997, *S. pyogenes* resistance to macrolides rose from 1.7 % of strains tested to 43 % of strains [10]. About 12 % of healthy children tested were carriers of *S. pyogenes* and 38 % of them were carrying a macrolide-resistant strain [11].

An in-vitro study [12] showed that *S. pyogenes* was susceptible to moxifloxacin, with a MIC$_{90}$ of 0.12 µg/mL (see Table 3). Thus, moxifloxacin could be considered as an alternative in the treatment of *S. pyogenes* infections. In addition, due to the high rate of macrolide resistance in some countries, moxifloxacin could be a good option for treatment of Group A Streptococcus-related diseases for those adult patients with allergy to beta-lactams.

Conclusion

Moxifloxacin has improved anti-Gram-positive activity in comparison to previous fluoroquinolones, especially against methicillin-susceptible and resistant *Staphylococcus aureus* (MSSA, MRSA), vancomycin-sensitive and resistant enterococci (VSE, VRE) and macrolide-resistant Group A beta-haemolytic

Streptococcus (MacR GABHS). Moxifloxacin provides clinicians with another therapeutic option for those difficult-to-treat infections when the spectrum of conventional antibiotics is compromised due to resistance or if the patient cannot tolerate the usual first-line agents.

References

1. Fine MJ et al. (1994) Efficacy of pneumococcal vaccination in adults, a meta-analysis of randomized controlled trials. Archives of Internal Medicine 154(23):2666–2677
2. Pittet D, Wenzel RP (1995) Nosocomial bloodstream infections. Archives of Internal Medicine 155:27–334
3. Hughes JM, Tenover FC (1997) Approaches to limiting emergence of antimicrobial resistance in bacteria in human populations. Clinical Infectious Diseases 24(suppl. 1):S131–135
4. Handwerger S, Raucher R, Altarac D et al. (1993) Nosocomial outbreak due to Enterococcus faecium highly resistant to vancomycin, penicillin and gentamicin. Clinical Infectious Diseases 16:750–755
5. Panillo AL, Culver DH, Gaynes RP et al. (1992) Methicillin resistant Staphylococcus aureus in US hospitals, 1975–1991. Infection Control and Hospital Epidemiology 13:582–586
6. Malathum K, Singh KV, Murray BE (1998) In vitro activity of moxifloxacin against gram-positive bacteria. In: Interscience Conference of Antimicrobial Agents and Chemotherapy, 1998, Abstract E204
7. Woodcock JM, Andrews JM, Boswell FJ, Brenwald NP, Wise R (1997) In vitro activity of BAY 12-8039, a new fluoroquinolone. Antimicrobial Agents and Chemotherapy 41(1):101–106
8. von Eiff C, Peters G (1998) Comparative in vitro activity of moxifloxacin, trovafloxacin and quinupristin-dalfopristin against staphylococci. In: Interscience Conference of Antimicrobial Agents and Chemotherapy, 1993, Abstract E212a
9. McMillan JA, Sandstrom C, Weiner LB et al. (1986) Viral and bacterial organisms associated with acute pharyngitis in a school-aged population. Journal of Pediatrics 109:747–752
10. Esposito S, Noviello S, Ianniello F, D'Errico G (1997) Epidemiological survey of erythromycin-resistance in S. pyogenes in Italy. In: Interscience Conference of Antimicrobial Agents and Chemotherapy, Abstract E111
11. Esposito S. Unpublished data
12. Esposito S, Noviello S, Ianniello F (1998) In vitro activity of moxifloxaxin compare with other fluoroquinolones against different erythromycin-resistant phenotypes of group A β-hemolytic streptococcus. In: Interscience Conference of Antimicrobial Agents and Chemotherapy 1998, Abstract E193

Chapter 6

Pre-clinical Microbiology – Atypical Organisms   6

Cécile M. Bébéar

Abstract. The in-vitro activity of moxifloxacin was reviewed and compared to other fluoro-quinolones, macrolides, and tetracyclines against atypical and intracellular organisms such as *Mycoplasma, Chlamydia* and *Legionella* spp. Moxifloxacin at 0.25 µg/mL inhibited 100% of all the mycoplasma strains tested. All *Chlamydia pneumoniae* strains were inhibited between 0.06 and 1 µg/mL. Moxifloxacin was very effective against *Legionella pneumophila* with a MIC of 0.06 µg/mL. The MBC values of moxifloxacin against *Mycoplasma pneumoniae* and *Chlamydia pneumoniae* were equal to or within one dilution step of the MIC values. Moxifloxacin was effective in eliminating *M. pneumoniae* and *C. pneumoniae* from the lungs of animal models.

This chapter will focus on the three major atypical pathogens implicated in respiratory tract infections; these are *Mycoplasma pneumoniae, Chlamydia pneumoniae* and *Legionella pneumophila*.

M. pneumoniae and *C. pneumoniae* are responsible for 15 to 40% of community-acquired pneumonia and 6 to 15% of acute bronchitis [1, 2]. Because these pathogens are not expected to respond to standard empirical treatment, the choice of antimicrobial therapy for pneumonia is very important.

The atypical organisms are characterized by their location inside cells. Consequently, effective antimicrobials must have high intracellular activity against these pathogens. Moxifloxacin shows good penetration into human neutrophils and tissue-cultured epithelial cells have intracellular concentrations that are approximately 10 times higher than those found in extracellular fluid. Moxifloxacin is active against *Staphylococcus aureus* inside the neutrophils, thus suggesting good clinical potential against intracellular pathogens [3].

The penetration of moxifloxacin into alveolar macrophages has been measured and compared to serum concentrations. Macrophage concentrations were found to be 20 to 90-fold higher than serum concentrations, thus exceeding the MIC_{90} of respiratory tract pathogens such as *Streptococcus pneumoniae, Haemophilus influenzae,* and the atypical pathogens such as *M. pneumoniae, C. pneumoniae* and *L. pneumophila* [4].

Investigating the activity of moxifloxacin against mycoplasma in more detail; mycoplasma lack cell walls, thus there are only three classes of antibiotics which are available for their treatment: tetracyclines, macrolides and fluoroquinolones. Table 1 shows the different species of *Mycoplasma* and the MIC_{90} and MBC values obtained for moxifloxacin, ofloxacin, doxycycline, and erythromycin [5]. Moxifloxacin showed excellent activity against *M. pneumoniae*, with a MIC_{90} value of 0.12 µg/mL, ten-fold lower than that of ofloxacin and equivalent to that

Table 1
Susceptibility of *Mycoplasma* spp. to moxifloxacin and selected antibiotics

Organism	MIC$_{90}$	MBC
	(µg/mL)	(µg/mL)
M. pneumoniae		
Moxifloxacin	0.12	0.25
Ofloxacin	1	4
Doxycycline	0.12	8
Erythromycin	≤0.015	ND
M. genitalium		
Moxifloxacin	0.03	0.25
Ofloxacin	1	4
Doxycycline	0.06	4
Erythromycin	≤0.015	ND
M. hominis		
Moxifloxacin	0.06	0.25
Ofloxacin	0.5	2
Doxycycline	0.03	2
Erythromycin	>32	ND
U. urealyticum		
Moxifloxacin	0.25	1
Ofloxacin	4	8
Doxycycline	0.5	16
Erythromycin	1	ND

of doxycycline. Differences between these antibiotics were even more pronounced for minimum bactericidal concentration (MBC) values. For moxifloxacin the MBC value was close to the MIC value with a difference of only one dilution (0.12 vs. 0.25 µg/mL). This was not the case for ofloxacin (1 vs. 4 µg/mL) or doxycycline (0.12 vs. 8 µg/mL). Against *Mycoplasma genitalium*, a genital mycoplasma, moxifloxacin showed improved activity with a MIC$_{90}$ value of 0.03 µg/mL and a correspondingly better bactericidal effect.

Among the other genital mycoplasmas, such as *Mycoplasma hominis* and *Ureaplasma urealyticum*, moxifloxacin showed activity comparable to that of doxycycline with a MIC$_{90}$ value of 0.06 µg/mL for *M. hominis* and 0.25 µg/mL for *U. urealyticum*. Moxifloxacin had a significant bactericidal effect against both pathogens [5].

The in-vitro activity of moxifloxacin has been investigated using animal models. One study used guinea pigs infected intranasally with *M. pneumoniae* and administered 1, 3 or 10 mg/kg moxifloxacin over six days. Moxifloxacin eradicated *M. pneumoniae* in lungs as demonstrated by both culture and PCR (polymerase chain reaction) methods [6].

There are few antimicrobials available for the treatment of chlamydial infections. Data from three studies [7–9] compared the activity of moxifloxacin against *C. pneumoniae* with these antimicrobials. Results are tabulated in Table 2. The first study showed good activity of moxifloxacin compared to ciprofloxacin and erythromycin. Moxifloxacin's MIC$_{90}$ value was 0.06 µg/mL, >30 times lower

Table 2
Three studies comparing the susceptibility of *Chlamydia* spp. to moxifloxacin and selected antibiotics

Organism	MIC$_{90}$ (µg/mL)	MBC (µg/mL)
C. pneumoniae		
Moxifloxacin[a]	0.06	0.06
Ciprofloxacin[a]	2	2
Erythromycin[a]	0.25	0.5
Moxifloxacin[b]	0.06	0.125
Minocycline[b]	0.06	0.125
Moxifloxacin[c]	1	1
Ofloxacin[c]	1	1
Doxycycline[c]	0.25	0.25
Erythromycin[c]	0.125	0.25
C. trachomatis[a,b]		
Moxifloxacin	0.06	0.06
Ciprofloxacin	2	2
Minocycline	0.03	0.06
Erythromycin	0.25	0.5
C. psittaci[a,b]		
Moxifloxacin	0.06	0.06
Minocycline	0.06	0.125

[a] Woodcock et al. 1997.
[b] Donati et al. 1997.
[c] Roblin et al. 1998.

than that of ciprofloxacin and > 4 times lower than that of erythromycin. In the second study, there was also good activity of moxifloxacin, comparable to that of minocycline. On the other hand, the third study obtained a MIC$_{90}$ value for moxifloxacin against *C. pneumoniae* of about 1 µg/mL, which was 10 times higher than previously described values. The same study reported the activity of doxycycline as 0.25 µg/mL and erythromycin as 0.125 µg/mL. These discrepancies may be due to differences in methods, especially in the type of cell used for the *Chlamydia* culture. It was noteworthy that in all studies MBC values were equivalent to MIC values against *C. pneumoniae*.

Moxifloxacin showed good activity against other species of *Chlamydia*, e.g. *C. trachomatis*, a genital species, and *C. psittaci*, an animal species. Moxifloxacin activity was comparable to that of minocycline with a MIC$_{90}$ value of 0.06 µg/mL. Again, moxifloxacin MBC values were equal to MIC values [7, 8].

Animal models have also been described for *Chlamydia* and moxifloxacin. In one study [10], mice were infected intranasally with *C. pneumoniae* and treated orally with moxifloxacin. Here again, moxifloxacin succeeded in eradicating *C. pneumoniae* in lungs with negative culture.

The last atypical species to be discussed is *Legionella pneumophila*. Unlike *Mycoplasma* and *Chlamydia*, *Legionella* infections largely remain a hospital issue with only a small array of antimicrobials available for their treatment: erythromycin and other macrolides, rifampin and the fluoroquinolones. Table 3 compares moxifloxacin, erythromycin, rifampin and doxycycline activity against

Table 3
Susceptibility of *L. pneumo-phila* to moxifloxacin and selected antibiotics

L. pneumophila	MIC$_{90}$ (µg/mL)
Moxifloxacin	0.06
Erythromycin	0.12
Rifampin	0.008
Doxycycline	8

L. pneumophila. The data show that after rifampin (0.008 µg/mL), moxifloxacin had the best MIC$_{90}$ value at 0.06 g/mL [11].

The fluoroquinolones, pefloxacin, ciprofloxacin and sparfloxacin have shown inhibition of *L. pneumophila*'s growth in alveolar macrophages, and in animal models [11]. So, moxifloxacin may have a potential role in the treatment of *Legionella* infections in addition to other treatments.

Conclusion

In conclusion, moxifloxacin shows very promising in-vitro activity against atypical and intracellular pathogens involved in respiratory and genital tract infections. This new methoxyquinolone has bactericidal activity at therapeutic concentrations against these pathogens and its efficacy has been proven in animal models for *M. pneumoniae* and *C. pneumoniae*. Finally, moxifloxacin could be a good alternative against these microorganisms in macrolide-intolerant patients or in combination therapy in severe atypical infections e.g. Legionellas.

References

1. Mayaud C (1997) Epidémiologie des infections respiratoires basses de l'adulte – Rôle de Chlamydia pneumoniae et Mycoplasma pneumoniae. La Presse Médicale 26:1248–1253
2. Marston BJ et al. (1997) Incidence of community-acquired pneumonia requiring hospitalization. Archives of Internal Medicine 157:1709–1718
3. Pascuals A, Garcia I, Ballesta S, Perea EJ (1999) Uptake and intracellular activity of moxifloxacin in human neutrophils and tissue-cultured epithelial cells. Antimicrobial Agents and Chemotherapy 43:12–15
4. Andrews J, Honeybourne D, Jevons G, Wise R (1998) Penetration of moxifloxacin into bronchial mucosa, epithelial lining fluid and alveola macrophages following a single 400 mg oral dose. In: 38th International Congress of Antimicrobial Agents and Chemotherapy, 1998, Abstract A29
5. Bébéar CM, Renaudin H, Boudjadja A, Bébéar C (1998) In vitro activity of BAY 12-8039, a new fluoroquinolone against mycoplasmas. Antimicrobial Agents and Chemotherapy 42:703–704
6. Jacobs E, Dalhoff A, Brunner H (1996) Efficacy of BAY 12-8039 in *Mycoplasma pneumoniae* infected guinea pigs. In: 36th International Congress of Antimicrobial Agents and Chemotherapy, New Orleans. 1996, Abstract F17
7. Woodcock JM, Andrews JM, Boswell FJ, Brenwald NP, Wise R (1997) In vitro activity of BAY 12-8039, a new fluoroquinolone. Antimicrobial Agents and Chemotherapy, 41:101–106

8. Donati M, Rumpianesi F, Pava G, Sambri V, Cevenini R (1997) In vitro activity of BAY 12-8039 against Chlamydia trachomatis and Chlamydia pneumoniae. In: 37th International Congress of Antimicrobial Agents and Chemotherapy, Toronto, 1997, Abstract F142

9. Roblin PM, Hammerschlag MR (1998) In vitro activitiy of a new 8-methoxyquinolone, BAY 12-8039, against Chlamydia pneumoniae. Antimicrobial Agents and Chemotherapy 42:951–952

10. Waterbury K, Wang JJ, Barbiero M, Federici J, Ohlin C, Huguenel ED (1996) Efficacy of BAY 12-8039, a potent new quinolone, in mouse models of typical and atypical respiratory infection. In: 36th International Congress of Antimicrobial Agents and Chemotherapy, New Orleans, 1996, Abstract F18

11. Schulin T, Wennersten CB, Ferraro MJ, Moellering RC Jr, Eliopoulos GM (1998), Susceptibilities of Legionella spp. to newer antimicrobials in vitro. Antimicrobial Agents and Chemotherapy 42:1520–1523

CHAPTER 7

Pre-clinical Microbiology – Summary I

BERND WIEDEMANN

The previous chapters of pre-clinical microbiology are summarised. Dr. Haken-beck dealt mainly with the problems concerning *Streptococcus pneumoniae*. She indicated that there now exist penicillin-resistant and even multi-drug resistant pneumococci. This resistance does not affect the activity of the new fluoro-quinolones, and moxifloxacin is especially active against these strains having MIC values ranging from 0.06 to 0.12 µg/mL. Additionally the various quin-olones appear to differ in their ability to select for resistance development, so care must still be taken when treating respiratory tract infections with these drugs.

Dr. Esposito discussed Gram-positive cocci and *Streptococcus pyogenes* in particular. Moxifloxacin may be an alternative to macrolide antibiotics as *S. pyo-genes* macrolide resistance is increasing. With regard to *Staphylococcus aureus*, there is sensitivity to moxifloxacin, but care must be taken with methicillin-resistant strains. It is not yet certain whether moxifloxacin should be used as a first, second, or third-line drug for these pathogens or indeed at all. This point will need further discussion.

In terms of enterococci, not all are sensitive to moxifloxacin, but *Enterococcus faecalis* and especially vancomycin-resistant enterococci show variable sensitivi-ty to moxifloxacin, however, caution must be exercised with all quinolones as therapeutic agents for enterococci.

Atypical organisms were covered by Dr. Bébéar. She explained that moxifloxa-cin is especially active against those organisms which cause respiratory tract infections. Moxifloxacin achieves concentrations well in excess of MIC values, it kills *Chlamydia*, *Mycoplasma* and *Legionella*, and it is effective in animal models.

The second section of the Pre-clinical Microbiology will deal with other in-vitro aspects of moxifloxacin.

CHAPTER 8

Pre-clinical Microbiology – Mycobacteria   8

STEPHEN H. GILLESPIE

Abstract. Mycobacterial diseases pose a significant threat to public health. The incidence of tuberculosis is increasing worldwide. Primary multiple-drug resistance is also rising and has reached almost 15% in some countries. There have been no new anti-tuberculosis agents introduced since rifampicin in the 1960s. Quinolones have been proposed as potential new antimycobacterial agents. They have several characteristics which suggest this role: potent activity against many species of mycobacteria, wide tissue penetration and distribution within macrophages. There have been a few clinical trials of quinolones in treating tuberculosis, and studies with ciprofloxacin show promising early bactericidal activity.

Moxifloxacin has potent activity against the mycobacteria causing human disease. Studies in mice confirm the activity *in vivo*. Further studies of the activity of moxifloxacin in anti-mycobacterial therapy should be undertaken.

Introduction

The incidence of tuberculosis is rising worldwide and resistance to anti-tuberculosis agents is also on the increase. Multiple-drug resistant tuberculosis (MDRTB), with resistance to both isoniazid and rifampicin, is becoming more prevalent. Today there are an estimated 50 million people infected, with very high rates in countries with poor control mechanisms. In Latvia, for instance, up to 14.4% of tuberculosis cases show primary drug resistance and 30% of all tuberculosis in that country is multidrug-resistant [1]. The prevalence of MDRTB is set to rise throughout the world.

The purpose of this chapter is to determine whether moxifloxacin has the potential to be a useful anti-mycobacterial agent that could be used as part of the treatment of tuberculosis.

Results and Discussion

In order to be an effective anti-tuberculosis agent, moxifloxacin must be able to reach its target. Mycobacteria are located inside macrophages, in solid caseous foci, in cavities and bronchii. Moxifloxacin shows good penetration into these sites, as will be demonstrated in later chapters.

Antimycobacterial agents must have excellent early bactericidal activity, that is the ability to kill organisms quickly and to reduce total bacterial number. They must also have good sterilising activity, meaning the ability to kill the organisms that are metabolizing very slowly and are responsible for relapses. In addition, the agent should prevent the emergence of resistance, which has proved to be such a problem of late in tuberculosis therapy.

Quinolones are good anti-mycobacterial or anti-tuberculosis agents because they are bactericidal, they have good tissue penetration, they acccumulate within the macrophage and some appear to be safe in long-term use. There are many ways of evaluating anti-tuberculosis agents, these include in-vitro studies (using MIC), in-vivo studies in mice, and clinical trials, either early bactericidal (Phase II) trials or controlled comparative clinical trials (Phase III). This chapter will refer principally to in-vitro and in-vivo mice studies because few comparative clinical trials have been performed.

A comparative trial of ciprofloxacin in the treatment of tuberculosis, showed that a drug regimen of isoniazid, rifampicin and ciprofloxacin, was as effective as the standard regimen in patients who were HIV sero-negative [2]. The trial demonstrated that ciprofloxacin lacked bactericidal activity in those patients who were HIV sero-positive. It is hoped that moxifloxacin, as part of an alternative combination regimen, might prove to be more effective in these patients.

Table 1 summarizes the results of in-vitro studies which compared the activity of fluoroquinolones against *Mycobacterium tuberculosis* (TB). The studies revealed that trovafloxacin did not have useful anti-mycobacterial activity (MIC$_{90}$ vs. TB > 8 µg/mL) [3]. Other fluoroquinolones tested were grepafloxacin, which had a MIC$_{90}$ value vs. TB of 1 µg/mL [4], and sparfloxacin which had a MIC$_{90}$ value of approximately 0.25 µg/mL [5]. Moxifloxacin appears to be a

Table 1. The in-vitro activity of fluoroquinolones against *M. tuberculosis*. Moxi – moxifloxacin; Spar – sparfloxacin; Levo – levofloxacin; Trova- trovafloxacin; Grepa – grepafloxacin

Study	Activity MIC$_{90}$ µg/mL					
	n	Moxi	Spar	Levo	Trova	Grepa
Felmingham (1997)[a]	33	–	–	–	32	–
Yew (1994)[a]	39(S)	–	0.06	0.25	–	–
	42(R)	–	0.125	0.25	–	–
Ji (1995)[d]	18	–	0.5	1.0	–	–
Ji (1998)[d]	20	0.25–0.5	0.5	–	–	–
Felmingham (1997b)[d]	25	0.25	–	–	–	–
Gross (1997)[b]	107	0.5	–	–	–	–
Gillespie (1999)[b]	19	0.25	>0.25	>0.25	–	–
Hoffner (1997)[c]	23	–	≤1.0	1.0	≥8.0	–
Vacher (1997)[b]	33	–	–	–	–	1.0

MIC determinations:
[a] Broth dilution.
[b] Proportion method.
[c] Bactec method.
[d] Agar dilution (S) sensitive (R) resistant to 3 first-line drugs.

Table 2. The activity of fluoroquinolones in mouse infections of tuberculosis

Study	Compound	Dose[a] mg/kg/day	Summary of main results
Chadwick (1989)	Ciprofloxacin		Reduction in cfu. Liver and spleen
Truffot-Permot (1991)	Pefloxacin	50	Inactive
	Ofloxacin	300 and 150	Improved survival, reduction in cfu.
Klemens (1994)	Levofloxacin	100 and 200	Reduction in cfu. Spleen and lung
	Ofloxacin	200 and 300	Slightly less active than levofloxacin
	Sparfloxacin	50 and 100	Most active compound
Ji (1991)	Ofloxacin	100–300	Less active at 300 than sparfloxacin
	Sparfloxacin	12.5–100	Improved survival, reduction in lung lesions and spleen weight
Ji (1995)	Levofloxacin	50–300	More active than ofloxacin
	Ofloxacin	150–300	Only moderately active at top dose
	Sparfloxacin	50–100	Most active (100 = 300) levofloxacin[b]
Lalande (1993)	Ofloxacin	300	Active, but less so than sparfloxacin
	Sparfloxacin	100 and 50	Reduction in cfu. and weight; spleens and lungs
Ji (1998)	Ciprofloxacin	15–100	No activity
	Sparfloxacin	25–100	Improved survival, reduction in lung lesions and spleen weight
	Moxifloxacin	25–100	More bacterial than sparfloxacin
Miyazaki (1998)	Moxifloxacin	20 and 100	Reduction in spleen cfu. and spleen lung weights

[a] In some experiments was for 6 days weekly.
[b] Activity assessed on survival, reduction in spleen weights/lung lesions and cfu.

potential anti-mycobacterial, with a MIC_{90} value against *M. tuberculosis* of 0.25 μg/mL [5]. These values are supported by a number of researchers who found the moxifloxacin MIC_{90} vs. TB to be in the same range [6–8].

Based on in-vivo mouse studies (Table 2), sparfloxacin appeared to be the most effective anti-tuberculosis agent with significant bactericidal efficacy [9–12]. More recent studies, however, indicated that moxifloxacin was more bactericidal against TB than sparfloxacin in the mouse model [13]. This is very encouraging information and suggests that moxifloxacin is active in vivo.

With more immunocompromised patients, the atypical mycobacteria are becoming a common clinical problem and fluoroquinolones such as moxifloxacin may have a role to play here as well. In-vitro data [4, 5, 8, 14, 15] showed that moxifloxacin had very good activity against *Mycobacterium avium-intracellulare*, which is a particularly difficult organism *to* treat (Table 3). Against *Mycobacterium kansasii* [4, 5, 8, 15], moxifloxacin showed good activity with a MIC_{90} value of 0.06 μg/mL, a little better than sparfloxacin, much better than grepafloxacin and even better than clinafloxacin and levofloxacin (Table 4). Of all the currently available new fluoroquinolones tested against *Mycobacterium*

Table 3. The in-vitro activity of fluoroquinolones against *M. avium-intracellulare*

Study	Activity MIC$_{90}$ µg/mL					
	n	Moxi	Spar	Clin	Levo	Grepa
Gillespie (1999)	10	1.0	1.0			-
Gross (1997)	10	>2[a]	-			-
Guillemin (1998)	-	2.0	4.0		8.0	-
Felmingham (1997)	28	4.0	-	-	-	-
Yew (1994)	25	-	8.0	>8.0	>8.0	-
Vacher (1997)	41	-	-			16

[a] Range of MICs 1 − >2 mg/L.

Table 4. The in-vitro activity of fluoroquinolones against *M. kansasii*

Study	Activity MIC$_{90}$ µg/mL					
	n	Moxi	Spar	Clin	Levo	Grepa
Gillespie (1999)	10	0.06	0.12			0.5
Gross (1997)	11	0.125	-	-	-	-
Yew (1994)	20	-	2.0	>8.0	4.0	-
Vacher (1997)	17	-	-			2.0

Moxi – moxifloxacin; Spar – sparfloxacin; Clin – clinafloxacin; Levo – levofloxacin; Grepa – grepafloxacin.

fortuitum, moxifloxacin again seemed to be the most active [4, 5, 8, 15]. Thus moxifloxacin shows good potential against the atypical mycobacteria.

One of the problems of anti-tuberculosis therapy is that patients often have very little capacity to resist the infection. Thus, the antimicrobial agent must do most of the work. This is particularly true for HIV sero-positive patients. To date, most of the data collected are MIC values which show that the fluoro-quinolones are very inhibitory against mycobacteria. The question is whether they are bactericidal.

The bactericidal activity of quinolones was investigated using *Mycoplasma fortuitum* as a model system due to its short incubation period [16]. Several measures were used including optimal bactericidal concentration. Preliminary data from these studies indicate that, of the four quinolones tested, moxifloxacin, sparfloxacin, ofloxacin and ciprofloxacin, moxifloxacin has the most potent bactericidal activity.

Conclusion

In summary, three fluoroquinolones appear to have anti-mycobacterial properties. Ciprofloxacin has been shown in clinical trials to be effective against mycobateria. It is bactericidal, it penetrates into tissues and macrophages, and long-term studies have shown it to be a very safe antimicrobial. An alternative to ciprofloxacin, sparfloxacin, is bacteriostatic, though recent data suggest it may not be bactericidal. Sparfloxacin has similar tissue and macrophage penetration characteristics to ciprofloxacin, but there are doubts regarding safety due to phototoxicity. This would limit use in the treatment of tuberculosis. Moxifloxacin is by far the most bactericidal of the fluoroquinolones against mycobacteria. It has similar pharmacokinetic characteristics to the other fluoroquinolones, with good tissue and macrophage penetration. Long-term safety data are awaited, and if the early data are borne out, moxifloxacin may well be an exciting new addition in the treatment of mycobacterial disease.

References

1. The WHO/IUATLD Anti-tuberculosis drug resistance in the world. World Health Organization, Geneva, 1997
2. Kennedy N, Berger L, Curram J et al. (1996) Randomized controlled trial of a drug regimen that includes ciprofloxacin for the treatment of pulmonary tuberculosis. Clinical Infectious Diseases 22:827–833
3. Hoffner SH, Gezelius L, Olsson-Liljequist B, (1997) In vitro activity of fluorinated quinolones and macrolides against drug resistant *Mycobacterium tuberculosis*. Journal of Antimicrobial Chemotherapy, 40:885–888
4. Vacher S, Maugein T, Leblanc F, Fourche J, Pellegrin JL (1997) Comparative antimycobacterial activity of three fluoroquinolones. In: Programme and abstracts of the 8th International Congress of Infectious Diseases, Boston, 1997, Abstract No. 10987
5. Gillespie SH, Billington O (1999) Activity of moxifloxacin against *Mycobacterium* sp. Journal of Antimicrobial Chemotherapy (in press)
6. Ji B, Loumis N, Maslo C, Truffot-Pernot C, Bonnafous P, Grosset J (1998). In vitro and in vivo activities of moxifloxacin and clinafloxacin against *Mycobacterium tuberculosis*. Antimicrobial Agents and Chemotherapy 42:2060–2069
7. Felmingham D, Robbins MJ, Leakey A, Salman H, Deacer C, Clark S et al. (1997) In vitro activity of BAY 12-8039. Poster No. 1156. In: Programme and Abstracts of the 8th European Conference of Clinical Microbiology and Infectious Diseases (ECCMID), Lausanne, 1997
8. Gross WM, Vadney FS, Ladutko I, Bonato DA, Campbell S (1997) In vitro activity of Bay 12-8039: a new methoxyquinolone against mycobacteria. In: Programme and Abstracts of the 37th International Congress of Antimicrobial Agents and Chemotherapy, Toronto, 1997. Abstract No. F144
9. Ji B, Truffot-Pernot C, Grosset J (1991) In vitro and in vivo activities of sparfloxacin (AT-4140) against *Mycobacterium tuberculosis*. Tubercle 72:181–186
10. Ji B, Lounis N, Truffot-Pernot C, Grosset J (1995) In vitro and in vivo activities of levofloxacin against *Mycobacterium tuberculosis*. Antimicrobial Agents and Chemotherapy 39:1341–1344
11. Klemens SP, Sharpe CA, Rogge MC, Cynamon MH (1994) Activity of levofloxacin in a murine model of tuberculosis. Antimicrobial Agents and Chemotherapy 38:1476–1479
12. Lalande V, Truffot-Pernot C, Paccaly-Moulin A, Grosset J, Ji B (1993) Powerful bactericidal activity of sparfloxacin (AT-4140) against *Mycobacterium tuberculosis* in mice. Antimicrobial Agents and Chemotherapy 37:407–413

13. Ji B, Lounis N, Masio C, Truffot-Pernot C, Bonnafous P, Grosset J (1998) In vitro and in vivo activities of moxifloxacin and clinafloxacin against *Mycobacterium tuberculosis*. Antimicrobial Agents and Chemotherapy. 42:2066–2069

14. Guillemin I, Camban E, Sougakoff W, Jarlier V (1998) Inhibitory effects of BAY 12-8039 on Mycobacterial gyrases. In: Programme and Abstracts of the 38th International Congress of Antimicrobial Agents and Chemotherapy, San Diego, 1997. Abstract No. C179

15. Yew WW, Piddock LJ, Li MS, Lyon D, Chan CY, Chang AF (1994) In-vitro activity of quinolones and macrolides against mycobacteria. Journal of Antimicrobial Chemotherapy 34:343–351

16. Gillespie SH – unpublished data

Discussion on Pre-clinical Microbiology – Mycobacterium

QUESTION: Dr. Gillespie, considering the last most important discovery in anti-tuberculosis drugs was Rifampin, and that was 30 years ago, do you consider animal experiments in infection to be useful? The second point concerns clinical trials because we have two difficulties. The first one is that we have many drug-resistant strains, especially in new cases of tuberculosis, and the second one is that it is impossible to use monotherapy in tuberculosis. What is your opinion about these two problems?

ANSWER: Two difficult questions; the first is a very interesting one. Everyone conducts mouse studies to see whether new agents are useful for the treatment of humans with tuberculosis, even though mice and humans are different in terms of tuberculosis. Mouse studies are, however, a useful pointer. Had we relied on them entirely, we would have missed the activity of Rifampin, for example, so they are not a very good model. Having proved safety in animals, I think it is much better to do studies in humans where the disease occurs and where conditions are different.

To answer the second point about clinical trials, perhaps I can pose a question. The problem with clinical trials is that there are new ideas about what we can do about the threat of tuberculosis in general, and drug-resistant tuberculosis in particular. Clearly, we can't use any agent as monotherapy but how are we going to evaluate a new therapy against tuberculosis after we have shown the organism is susceptible?

The usual protocol requires six months therapy which most people do not finish. How are we going to reduce that treatment time? We need new ideas and new drugs that are going to be more effective. We need to shorten therapy to ensure that more people complete treatment so that we get higher cure rates. That will protect against drug resistance. So is moxifloxacin going to be the agent that will shorten chemotherapy significantly thereby improving treatment?

CHAPTER 9

In-vitro Activity of Moxifloxacin [Bay 12-8039], an 8-methoxy Quinolone, Compared to Other Fluoroquinolones Against Anaerobic Bacteria

ELLIE GOLDSTEIN

Abstract. The in vitro activity of moxifloxacin [Bay 12-8039], a new 8-methoxy-quinolone, against anaerobic bacteria was reviewed and compared to that of other fluoroquinolones such as ciprofloxacin, levofloxacin, ofloxacin and sparfloxacin. Moxifloxacin has a broad spectrum of activity against anaerobic bacteria, usually has an MIC_{90} 2 µg/mL against most species, was more potent than levofloxacin and ciprofloxacin and was effective against most clinically important anaerobic pathogens. It had a similar spectrum of activity and MIC patterns in comparison with trovafloxacin. The fusobacteria were relatively resistant to all the fluoroquinolones. Extrapolating from the in vitro data, moxifloxacin may be effective against skin and soft tissue infections caused by human and animal bites, and has potential for clinical use in respiratory tract infection, abdominal surgical and gynaecological infections. Clinical evaluation in mixed aerobic/ anaerobic infections appears warranted.

Introduction

Moxifloxacin [Bay 12-8039] is a new 8-methoxyquinolone agent with once daily dosing which has not shown evidence of phototoxicity [10, 11]. Moxifloxacin possesses activity against aerobic Gram-positive and Gram-negative bacteria as well as anaerobes [4, 7, 8]. We review the literature on its activity against pathogenic anaerobic bacteria.

Results and Discussion

Six studies identified in the literature search [1, 2, 5, 7, 9, 13] varied as to media, method and inoculum used, as well as the numbers and ranges of isolates tested. Some of the studies speciated isolates while others grouped various species together or did not speciate the isolates of a specific genera. Some studies used small numbers of isolates (< 10) of a particular genus or species and therefore only MIC_{50} values were determined. Consequently, results from the various studies are not entirely comparable. Several studies were found in abstracts from meetings and manuscripts in submission from which full data could not be derived but which are cited for completeness [3, 6, 12].

Aldridge and Ashcraft [1] found 91 % of 410 anaerobes were susceptible to 2 µg/mL of moxifloxacin. They used a broth microdilution method and an inoculum of 10^5 cfu/mL. They felt that moxifloxacin was comparable to metronidazole and 16-fold more active than ciprofloxacin, ofloxacin, cefoxitin and cefotetan. An adapted summary of their data is listed in Table 1.

Bauernfeind [2] studied a limited number of anaerobes and used Wilkins Chalgren medium with 10% sheep blood and inoculum of 10^5 cfu/mL. The following MIC$_{90}$ values were reported: B. fragilis [20 strains], 2 µg/mL; Bacteroides spp. [6 isolates], 4 µg/mL; C. difficile [20 strains], 2 µg/mL; and Clostridium species [5 strains], 0.13 µg/mL. The MIC$_{90}$ values of clinafloxacin, gatifloxacin and trovafloxacin were within one doubling dilution of the moxifloxacin values; levofloxacin and ciprofloxacin were markedly less active.

Elund et al. [5] used PDM Antibiotic Sensitivity Medium supplemented with 5% defibrinated horse blood and an inoculum of 10^5 to 10^6 cfu/mL to study the activity of moxifloxacin and levofloxacin. Unfortunately, most isolates are not speciated and their specific clinical sources are not stated. Moxifloxacin had the following MIC$_{90}$ values: B. fragilis [50 strains], 1.0 µg/mL; Bacteroides spp, Porphyromonas spp, Prevotella spp [50 strains], 2.0 µg/mL; Clostridium difficile [50 strains], 2.0 µg/mL; C. perfringens [30 strains], 0.5 µg/mL; Fusobacterium spp. [50 strains], 0.25 µg/mL; Peptostreptococcus spp. [50 strains], 1,0 µg/mL; and Propionibacterium acnes [30 strains], 0.25 µg/mL.

Goldstein et al. [7] studied the activity of moxifloxacin and the 11 comparator antimicrobials against anaerobes isolated from animal bite wounds in humans. They used Brucella blood agar supplemented with 5% sheep blood, hemin and vitamin K1 and an inoculum of 10^5 cfu/mL. A synopsis of the data is shown in Table 1. Moxifloxacin was active against almost all animal and human bite wound anaerobes which were susceptible to 0.5 µg/mL except for Fusobacterium nucleatum and other Fusobacterium species (MIC$_{90}$ of >4.0 µg/mL) and one strain of Prevotella loeschii (MIC of 2.0 µg/mL). In comparison, the other quinolones tested were less active than moxifloxacin against the anaerobes, including peptostreptococci and Porphyromonas. The fusobacteria were relatively resistant to all the fluoroquinolones tested. This study suggested that moxifloxacin was active in vitro against a wide variety of anaerobic bacteria that are encountered in human and animal bite infections.

MacGowan et al. [9] studied the comparative activity of moxifloxacin against 218 anaerobes using Wilkins Chalgren agar supplemented with 5% lysed horse blood and an inoculum of 10^4 cfu/mL. The MIC$_{90}$ for all 218 isolates was 2 µg/mL for moxifloxacin, 16 µg/mL for ciprofloxacin, 0.5 µg/mL for clinafloxacin, 8 µg/mL for ofloxacin, and 1 µg/mL for trovafloxacin. An adapted summary of the data is listed in Table 1.

Woodcock et al. [13] compared moxifloxacin to trovafloxacin, ciprofloxacin, cefpodoxime and amoxicillin-clavulanate against a limited number of general clinical anaerobic isolates. They utilised an agar dilution method with Wilkins Chalgren agar supplemented with 50 µg of 1-(4-nitrophenyl)-glycerol per mL and 5% horse blood and a final inoculum of 10^4 cfu/spot. All tested anaerobic strains were susceptible to 2 µg/mL of moxifloxacin. These included B. fragilis (25 strains), Prevotella spp (3 strains), peptostreptococci (20 strains), C. perfringens (10 strains) and C. difficile (10 strains).

Limited data from abstracts was available. Wexler et al. [12] tested 180 anaerobes isolated from pulmonary infections with an agar dilution method

Table 1. In vitro activity of moxifloxacin [Bay 12-8039] against anaerobic bacteria as published in six studies

Organism	Ref/[No. isolates]	MIC$_{50/90}$ (µg/mL)			
		Moxi	Trova	Gati	Clina
Actinomyces spp.	9 [5]	0.003/–	1/–		0.25/–
Bacteroides spp. [unspecified]	2 [6]	0.5/–	0.5/–	0.5/–	0.5/–
Bacteroides capillosus	9 [9]	0.25/–	0.25/–		2
Bacteroides fragilis	1 [126]	0.5/2			
	2 [20]	1/2	0.5/1	0.5/1	0.5/2
	5 [50]	0.5/1			
	9 [10]	0.25/2	0.25/1		0.1/0.25
	13 [25]	0.25/0.25	1/1		
Bacteroides thetaiotaomicron	1 [35]	2/16			
	9 [11]	1/2	0.5/0.5		0.1/0.25
Bacteroides distasonis	1 [25]	0.5/2			
	9 [9]	1	0.5/–		0.1/–
Bacteroides ovatus	1 [25]	2/4			
	9 [14]	2/2	0.5/2		
Bacteroides vulgatus	1 [25]	0.5/2			
	9 [12]	0.5/2	0.25/0.5	0.25/2	0.2/0.25
Bacteroides uniformis	1 [14]	2/16			
	9 [6]	2/–	1/–		0.25/–
Bacteroides tectum	7 [22]	0.06/0.1			
Bifidobacterium spp.	9 [5]	1/–	1/–		0.25/–
Prevotella bivia	1 [21]	1/2			
Prevotella buccae	9 [5]	0.25/–	1/–		0.03/–
Prevotella disiens	1 [19]	0.5/0.5			
Prevotella heparinolytica	7 [12]	0.1/0.1			
Prevotella spp. [unspecified]	7 [26]	0.25/0.5			
Porphyromonas salivosa	7 [11]	0.1/0.1			
Porphyromonas gingivalis	7 [10]	0.06/0.06			
Porphyromonas spp. other	7 [14]	0.25/0.5			
Fusobacterium nucleatum	7 [21]	1/4			
	9 [7]	0.06/–	0.25/–		0.25/–
Fusobacterium spp.	1 [23]	0.1/0.5			
	5 [50]	0.1/0.25			
	7 [15]	4/8			
Clostridium perfringens	1 [20]	0.25/0.5			
	5 [30]	0.5/0.5			
	9 [6]	0.25/–	0.06/–		0.5/–
	13 [10]	0.5/0.5	0.5/1		

Table 1 (continued)

Organism	Ref/[No. isolates]	MIC$_{50/90}$ (µg/mL)			
		Moxi	Trova	Gati	Clina
Clostridium difficile	2 [20]	1/2	0.1/0.5	0.25/0.5	0.5/2
	5 [50]	2/2			
	13 [10]	1/2	2/2		
Clostridium ramosum	9 [5]	1/–	0.5/–		0.5/–
Clostridium spp.	1 [20]	0.25/1			
	2 [5]	0.07/–	0.1/–	0.25/–	0.06/–
	9 [14]	0.5/4	0.25/1		0.06/0.5
Eubacterium spp.	1 [14]	0.1/0.25			
	9 [7]	0.25/–	0.1/–		0.06/–
Lactobacillus spp.	9 [10]	0.25/0.5	0.25/0.5		0.1/0.25
Peptostreptococcus spp. [unspecified]	1 [25]	0.06/0.25			
	5 [50]	0.25/1			
	7 [9]	0.25/–			
	13 [20]	0.1//1	0.5/1		
Peptostreptococcus anaerobius	9 [5]	0.25/–	0.1/–		0.06/–
Peptostreptococcus asaccharolyticus	9 [5]	0.5/–	0.5/–		0.1/–
Peptrostreptococcus magnus	9 [27]	0.06/0.25	0.06/0.25		0.03/0.06
Peptostreptococcus micros	9 [5]	0.1/–	0.03/–		0.01/–
Propionibacterium acnes	5 [30]	0.1/0.25			
	9 [7]	0.25/–	1/–		0.06/–
Veillonella parvula	1 [18]	0.06/0.25			
	9 [10]	0.25/0.25	0.5/0.5		0.03/0.03

Moxi – moxifoxacin, Trova – trovafloxacin, Gati – gatifloxacin, Clina – clinafloxacin.

using Brucella 5% laked blood agar and an inoculum of 10^5 cfu/spot. Most (97%) of the isolates were susceptible to 2 µg/mL of moxifloxacin or trovafloxacin. The geometric mean MIC of *B. fragilis* isolates to moxifloxacin was 0.5 µg/mL and for *B. fragilis* group species it was 0.8 µg/mL. All the 18 *F. nucleatum* strains tested were susceptible to 0.25 µg/mL of moxifloxacin and "other" Fusobacterium strains to 0.5 µg/mL. This contrasts another study [7] which found higher MIC values for all fusobacteria.

Betriu et al. [3] reported that moxifloxacin "inhibited 80% and 94% of [218 strains] *B. fragilis* group strains at concentrations of 1 and 4 µg/mL, respectively." The non-*fragilis* members of the *B. fragilis* group were slightly less susceptible with the following MIC 90 values: *B. fragilis*, 1 µg/mL; *B. thetaiotaomicron*, 8 µg/mL; *B. uniformis*, 4 µg/mL. They concluded that moxifloxacin has a potential "role in treating mixed anaerobic infections caused by the *B. fragilis* group."

Conclusion

Overall, these studies demonstrate that moxifloxacin has a broad spectrum of in-vitro activity against anaerobic bacteria, usually has an $MIC_{90} = 2$ µg/mL against most species, is more potent than levofloxacin and ciprofloxacin against anaerobes, is effective against most clinically important anaerobes, would be effective against skin and soft tissue infections caused by human and animal bites and has potential for clinical use in respiratory tact infection, abdominal surgical infections and gynaecological infections. Clinical evaluation of its use in mixed aerobic/ anaerobic infections is warranted.

References

1. Aldridge KE, Ashcraft DS (1997) Comparison of the in vitro activities of Bay 12-8039, a new quinolone, and other antimicrobials against clinically important anaerobes. Antimicrob Agents Chemother 41:709–711
2. Bauernfeind A (1997) Comparison of the antibacterial activities of the quinolones Bay 12-8039, gatifloxacin, (Am-1155), trovafloxacin, clinafloxacin, levofloxacin and ciprofloxacin. J Antimicrob Chemother 40:639–651
3. Betriu C, Gomez M, Palau ML, Sanchez A, Picazo JJ (1998) In vitro activity of a new fluoroquinolone, Bay 12-8039, against *Bacteroides fragilis* group. Proceedings of the 38th Interscience Conference on Antimicrobial Agents and Chemotherapy. San Diego 24–27 September 1998, Abstract No. E-205, pg 228
4. Dalhoff A, Fischer E, Heidmann M, Hesse D. In vitro activity of Bay-12-8039, a new 8-methoxy-quinolone. Chemotherapy (Basel), In Press
5. Elund C, Sabouri S, Nord CE (1998) Comparative in vitro activity of Bay 12-8039 and five other antimicrobial agents against anarobic bacteria. Eur J Clin Microbiol Infect Dis. 17:193–195
6. Felmingham D, Robbins MJ, Leakey A, Salman H, Dencer C, Clark S, Ridgway GL, Gruneberg RN (1996) In vitro activity of Bay 12-8039 against bacterial respiratory tract pathogens, mycoplasmas and obligate anaerobic bacteria. Proceedings of the 36th Interscience Conference on Antimicrobial Agents and Chemotherapy. New Orleans 15–18 September 1996, Abstract No. F-8, p 101
7. Goldstein EJC, Citron DM, Hudspeth M, Gerardo SH, Merriam CV (1997) In vitro activity of Bay 12-8039, a new 8-methoxyquinolone, compared to the activities of 11 other antimicrobial agents against 390 aerobic and anaerobic bacteria isolated from human and animal bite wound skin and soft tissue infections in humans. Antimicrob Agents Chemother. 41:1552–1557
8. Herrington JA, Federici JA, Painter BG, Remy JM, Barbiero MI, Thurberg BE (1996) In vitro activity of Bay 12-8039, a new quinolone. Proceedings of the 36th Interscience Conference on Antimicrobial Agents and Chemotherapy. New Orleans 15–18 September 1996, Abstract No. F-4, p 100
9. MacGowan AP, Bowker KE, Holt HA, Wootton M, Reeves DS (1997) Bay 12-8039, a new 8-methoxy-quinolone: comparative in vitro activity with nine other antimicrobials against anaerobic bacteria. J Antimicrob Chemother 40:503–509
10. Petersen U, Bremm K-D, Dalhoff A, Endermann R, Heilmann W, Krebs A, Schenke T (1996) Synthesis and in vitro activity of Bay 12-8039, a new 8-methoxy-quinolone. Proceedings of the 36th Interscience Conference on Antimicrobial Agents and Chemotherapy. New Orleans 15–18 September 1996, Abstract No. F-1, p 100
11. Siefert HM, Domdey-Bette A, Henninger K, Hucke F, Kohlsdorfer C, Stass H (1996) Bay 12-8039, a new 8-methoxy-quinolone: comparison of the pharmacokinetics in different mammalian species. Proceedings of the 36th Interscience Conference on Antimicrobial Agents and Chemotherapy. New Orleans 15–18 September 1996, Abstract No. F-20, p 103

12. Wexler HM, Molitoris E, Finegold SM (1998) In vitro activity of moxifloxacin against anaerobic bacteria isolated from pulmonary specimens. Proceedings of the 38th Interscience Conference on Antimicrobial Agents and Chemotherapy. San Diego 24–27 September 1998, Abstract No. E-211, p 230
13. Woodcock JM, Andrews JM, Boswell FJ, Brenwald NP, Wise R (1997) In vitro activity of Bay 12-8039, a new fluoroquinolone. Antimicrob Agents Chemother 41:101–106

Discussion on Preclinical Microbiology – Anaerobes

QUESTION: Dr. Goldstein, most people agree that moxifloxacin has very good anaerobic activity. There are very high concentrations of moxifloxacin, both in the saliva and in the faeces. Despite that, we do not have any significant impact on either the pharyngeal or the intestinal microflora. Do you have an explanation for that?

ANSWER: This question has been discussed several times. We know that the quinolones are inactivated somewhat by the faeces. Another consideration is the inoculum effect. Let us suppose that there is a 99.9% kill rate and the pathogen load is 10^{11} microorganisms. With that kill rate, there is still 0.1% or 10^8 microorganisms remaining which is enough to repopulate the flora. So, there are some acute changes, but not enough to affect it ultimately. The oral flora exist in an environment with multiple structures and I suspect the same inoculum effect occurs there.

QUESTION: As a follow-up question, do you think that moxifloxacin is going to be as safe as ciprofloxacin especially in relation to *C. difficile* disease?

ANSWER: There is a perception that ciprofloxacin and the quinolones do not cause *C. difficile* disease. I think that the quinolones are relatively safe and will continue to be so, although I do not know of any correlation between MIC data and the development of *C. difficile* disease.

CHAPTER 10

Pre-clinical Microbiology – Fastidious Gram-negative Bacteria

ADOLF BAUERNFEIND

Abstract. The in-vitro activity of moxifloxacin against a group of fastidious bacterial pathogens was reviewed. Reports from different countries (USA, UK, Germany) were included. The activity (MIC) of moxifloxacin was compared to four other fluoroquinolones (ciprofloxacin, trovafloxacin, levofloxacin, grepafloxacin). Moxifloxacin and the other compounds were equipotent against the respiratory pathogens, *H. influenzae, H. parainfluenzae* and *M. catarrhalis* and *N. gonorrhoeae.* The maximum MIC_{90} was 0.13 µg/mL. *Pasteurella* spp. were most susceptible to the fluoroquinolones with maximum MIC_{90} of 0.06 µg/mL. Moxifloxacin was equally effective against ampicillin-resistant and ampicillin-susceptible strains of *H. influenzae* and *M. catarrhalis.* Macrolide resistance in *H. influenzae* produced a two-fold increase in the MICs of ciprofloxacin. A shift towards higher MICs of ciprofloxacin was observed in South Korea between 1993 and 1996 for *N. gonorrhoeae* within the susceptible and intermediate parts of the strain population. So far no trend to higher incidence of fluoroquinolone resistance has been observed among the fastidious pathogens included, in spite of extended use of fluoroquinolones in therapy of respiratory tract infections.

Introduction

This chapter will review the activity of fluoroquinolones against fastidious Gram-negative organisms, these include *Haemophilus influenzae, Haemophilus parainfluenzae* and *Moraxella catarrhalis*, which cause respiratory tract infections; *Neisseria gonorrhoeae*, which is involved in sexually transmitted diseases; *Neisseria meningitidis*, the causative organism for central nervous system infections and *Pasteurella* spp., which are found in skin and soft tissue infections. The fluoroquinolones that will be discussed are moxifloxacin, ciprofloxacin, trovafloxacin, levofloxacin and grepafloxacin. Each of these compounds is, or soon will be, available in most countries.

Results and Discussion

The data in Table 1 show the susceptibility of *H. influenzae* to the fluoroquinolones [1–3] and it is clear that there is no significant difference in the activity of these compounds. The data contain isolates from Germany, the United States, Spain and the United Kingdom and all were inhibited by 0.13 µg/mL. One strain of *H. influenzae* was recently reported [4] to be resistant to several fluoroquinolones and this may indicate a future problem.

Table 1. The comparative susceptibility of *H. influenzae* to fluoroquinolones

Compound	n	MICs (μg/mL)		
		Max. MIC$_{50}$	Max. MIC$_{90}$	Range
Moxifloxacin	748	0.03	0.06	0.008–0.13
Ciprofloxacin	748	0.03	0.03	0.004–0.03
Trovafloxacin	748	0.03	0.06	0.004–0.06
Levofloxacin	404	0.03	0.06	0.008–0.06
Grepafloxacin	308	0.03	0.06	n.a.

The major problem in treating infections due to *H. influenzae* was resistance to amino penicillins. The overall incidence of beta-lactamase producing strains from 30 reporting centres in the United States was 36%, ranging from 17–63%. The Alexander Study reported similar data for Europe, where the overall incidence was 28%, ranging from 5%–75%.

An important question is whether there is any correlation between resistance to ampicillin and susceptibility to quinolones. The answer is provided by the data in Fig. 1. Most strains of *H. influenzae* were susceptible to 0.06 μg/mL. This is independent of their resistance or susceptibility to ampicillin. The data is valid for all fluoroquinolones. So these agents provide a real alternative treatment.

Another problem with *H. influenzae* infections is macrolide resistance. Resistance to clarithromycin was defined as MIC >2 μg/mL and studies have shown [3] that

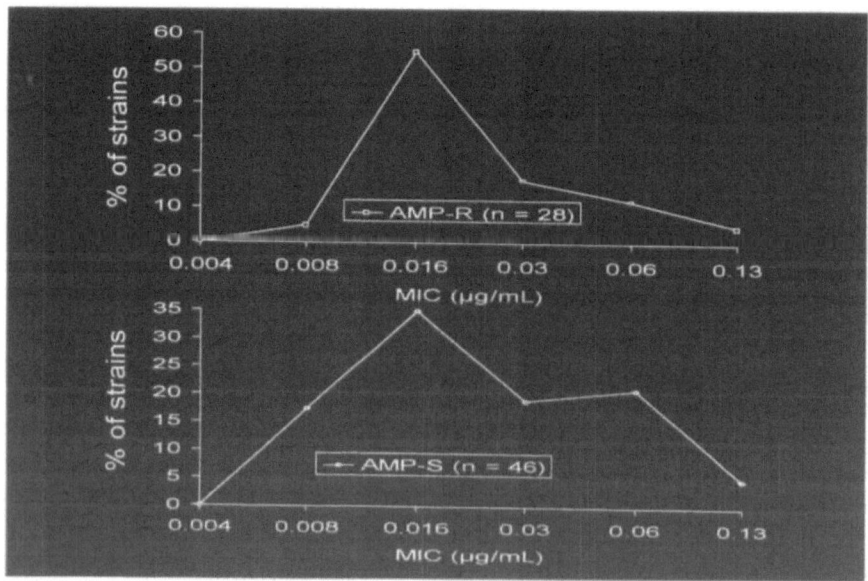

Fig. 1. The activity of moxifloxacin against ampicillin-resistant *H. influenzae*

resistant strains are less susceptible to ciprofloxacin by a factor of 2, i.e. 0.008 µg/mL rising to 0.016 µg/mL. *H. parainfluenzae* is becoming more accepted as causing respiratory tract infections. Studies on a small number (n = 11) of strains showed [1] moxifloxacin is about equiactive to the other fluoroquinolones that were evaluated. The MIC_{50} for moxifloxacin was 0.008 µg/mL and all strains were inhibited by 0.06 µg/mL.

    M. catarrhalis has a comparable susceptibility to the quinolones. More than 500 isolates from different countries were evaluated and all were inhibited by 0.13 µg/mL of moxifloxacin. At present, there are no reports of *M. catarrhalis* resistant to quinolones.

    One representative of the fastidious Gram-negative organisms in which resistance may be developing is *N. gonorrhoeae*. In general, it appeared to be very susceptible to fluoroquinolones. The MIC_{50} values for 68 isolates were comparable to those for respiratory pathogens. All strains were inhibited by 0.13 µg/mL of moxifloxacin and similar concentrations of the other quinolones. Nevertheless, a report by Lee and Chong [5] indicated a trend to resistance with strains in Korea having MICs of 1 µg/mL. The results are illustrated in Fig. 2 and compare the susceptibility of strains to ciprofloxacin in 1993 and 1996. While there was 4% resistant strains in 1993 and 2% in 1996, there was a concomitant decrease in susceptible strains and an increase in the intermediate resistant population. This shift from susceptible to intermediate populations would be missed if one focussed only on the resistant population.

    How does beta-lactamase production in *H. influenzae*, *M. catarrhalis* and *N. gonorrhoeae* influence their susceptibility to quinolones? Determination of the MIC values for moxifloxacin against either beta-lactamase positive or beta-lactamase negative isolates of those organisms showed no significant difference. The conclusion is that beta-lactamase production has no influence on susceptibility to quinolones.

    N. meningitidis attracted attention in Germany and other countries recently. Although some reports suggested there were resistant strains, to date all have been found to be highly susceptible to quinolones, $MIC_{90} < 0.006$ µg/mL.

    Many people suffer bites from animals or other humans. For example, it has been estimated that 50% of Americans are bitten during their lifetime. There is a broad spectrum of organisms that may be transferred by bites, including *Pasteurella* spp. The organisms are not cultured, not identified and no susceptibility testing is done,

Fig. 2
The susceptibility of
N. gonorrhoeae in South
Korea to ciprofloxacin

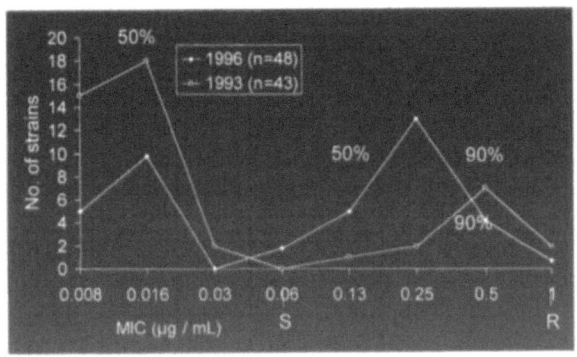

even though prophylaxis or treatment is necessary. Data published by Professor Goldstein [6] show that *Pasteurella* spp. are very susceptible to quinolones. The MIC_{50} against 55 strains of *Pasteurella* was 0.016 µg/mL and all strains were inhibited by 0.06 µg/mL.

Conclusion

The fastidious Gram-negative bacterial pathogens are among the most fluoroquinolone-susceptible pathogens. There is no remarkable difference in activity of quinolones against them. *Neisseria* spp. and *Pasteurella* spp. are more susceptible to fluoroquinolones than *Haemophilus spp* or *Moraxella* spp. Resistant mutants of *H. influenzae* and *N. gonorrhoeae* have been detected but, to date, their prevalence is very low.

References

1. Bauernfeind A (1997) Comparison of the antibacterial activities of the quinolones Bay 12-8039, gatifloxacin (AM 1155), trovafloxacin, clinafloxacin, levofloxacin and ciprofloxacin. Journal of Antimicrobial Chemotherapy 40:639–651
2. Woodcock JM, Andrews JM, Boswell FJ, Brenwald NP, Wise R (1997) In vitro activity of Bay 12-8039, a new fluoroquinolone. Antimicrobial Agents and Actions 41:101–106
3. Focht J (1998) In vitro activity of Bay 12-8039 compared with other fluoroquinolones against bacterial strains from upper and lower respiratory tract infections in general practice. In Programme and Abstracts of the Second European Congress of Chemotherapy, Hamburg, Germany 1998
4. Brueggemann AB, Kugler KC, Doern GV (1997) In vitro activity of Bay 12-8039, a novel 8-methoxyquinolone, compared to activities of six fluoroquinolones against *Streptococcus pneumoniae, Hemophilus influenzae,* and *Moraxella catarrhalis.* Antimicrobial Agents and chemotherapy 41:1594–1597
5. Lee K, Chong Y, Erdenschameg L, Song SS, Shin KH (1998) Incidence, epidemiology and evolution of reduced susceptibility to ciprofloxacin in Neisseria gonorrhoeae in Korea. Clinical Microbiology and Infection 627–633
6. Goldstein EJC, Citron DM, Hudspeth M, Gerardo SH, Merriam CV (1997) In vitro activity of Bay 12-8039, a new 8-methoxiquinolone, compared to the activities of 11 other oral antimicrobial agents against 390 aerobic and anaerobic bacteria isolated from human and animal bite wound skin and soft tissue infections in humans. Antimicrobial Agents and Chemotherapy 41:1552–1557

Discussion on Pre-clinical Microbiology – Fastidious Gram-negatives

QUESTION: I would be interested in the question of selection of resistance. Do you have experience about how many steps you need to select resistant organisms among anaerobes, mycobacteria and fastidious Gram-negative organisms?

ANSWER: We have some data on selection of resistance in *mycobacterium* for ciprofloxacin and mutation rates are less than 10^{-8} cfu/mL. We expect they will be even lower for moxifloxacin. The quinolones are very good at preventing the emergence of resistance in mycobacterial infections.

I do not know of any data or modeling for that in anaerobic bacteria. They have tended to be slower than other organisms to develop resistance, but some do, and there are certain strains that have innate resistance to some of the fluoroquinolones. The phenomenon is variable. We do not have experience in regional data on the selection of resistant mutants among the fastidious Gram-negative organisms.

The data on *Neisseria gonorrhoeae* are very interesting with regard to the last question. It shows that there are several components to resistance. One is the emergence of resistance and the other is the clonal spread of resistant strains. With the *N. gonorrhoeae*, it is quite clearly clonal spread in South Korea but in the rest of the world, that clone has not yet emerged. The resistance to quinolones of gonorrhoea is usually much less. The MIC_{90} for ciprofloxacin against *N. gonorrhoeae* is 0.12–0.25 µg/mL, so presumably the number of pre-existing resistant variants is very low.

We have looked for the number of pre-existing variants among the three respiratory pathogens, *S. pneumoniae, H. influenzae* and *M. catarrhalis*. These mutations are not induced, they occur spontaneously, so within any population you will find some. With pneumococcus and ciprofloxacin, it is very low, in the order of 10^{-10}. Over many years that pneumococcus has been exposed to ciprofloxacin, ofloxacin and norfloxacin, and other quinolones, it is quite remarkable that there are so few resistant pneumococci. With *H. influenzae* and *M. catarrhalis*, the selection rate is slightly higher, about 10^{-9}.

These rates of selection for resistant strains are much less than has been found for pneumococcus with other antimicrobials. This is quite good news, but we cannot foresee what is going to happen in the future, since we do not really know the complex interactions between the microbes in the upper respiratory tract. With *E. coli* we were quite sure that selection of resistance would be delayed or very few resistant strains would emerge. Now we see these resistant strains emerging and giving problems. It is necessary to be careful about resistance with all drugs, and especially with the new drugs, to maintain their clinical efficacy.

CHAPTER 11

Pre-clinical Microbiology –   **11**
Respiratory Tract Infections Susceptibility
Survey – USA

DANIEL SAHM

Abstract. Antimicrobial resistance among *Streptococcus pneumoniae* emphasizes the need for comprehensive and continued surveillance among respiratory bacterial pathogens. A centralised laboratory study was conducted in which *S. pneumoniae* (5,640 isolates), *Haemophilus influenzae* (6,588 isolates), and *Moraxella catarrhalis* (3,230 isolates) collected throughout the United States during the 1997–1998 respiratory season were tested using broth microdilution. Among *S. pneumoniae*, 64% were susceptible, 22% were intermediate, and 14% were resistant to penicillin. Depending on the geographic region examined, penicillin resistance ranged from 10% to 24%. Resistance to all antimicrobials tested (e.g. cephalosporins, macrolides, and trimethoprim-sulfamethoxazole) increased dramatically in the penicillin-resistant populations. Only the fluoroquinolones moxifloxacin (MIC$_{90}$, 0.25 µg/mL) and levofloxacin (MIC$_{90}$, 1 µg/mL) maintained high-level activity against all pneumococci. For *H. influenzae* and *M. catarrhalis*, 33% and 92% of the isolates, respectively, produced beta-lactamase. Resistance to agents other than ampicillin was uncommon among these species.

This report describes a study that was undertaken during the respiratory season 1997–1998 that encompassed approximately five months, and included strains collected from 373 geographically distributed institutions throughout the United States. Since there are approximately 6,000 institutions in the United States, this represents about 6 percent of the medical institutions. The strains were collected and tested in our laboratory using NCCLS methodology for *Haemophilus influenzae*, *Streptococcus pneumoniae* and *Moraxella catarrhalis*. The study tested 15,458 strains, 5,640 of which were *S. pneumoniae*, 6,588 *H. influenzae* and 3,230 *M. catarrhalis*.

Thirty three per cent of the *H. influenzae* strains examined were beta-lactamase positive. The resistance to amoxicillin/clavulanic acid and azithromycin was rare, at least in this collection of over 6,000 isolates. It was encountered in less than 0.1% of the strains tested. However, there was resistance to trimethoprim-sulfamethoxazole (TMP-SMX) of approximately 13%. No resistance to the newer or extended spectrum cephalosporins, either ceftriaxone or cefuroxime was encountered.

Ninety two percent of the *M. catarrhalis* strains that were isolated were beta-lactamase positive. However, there was discordance between beta-lactamase positive and resistance to ampicillin; only 82% of the strains were resistant as defined by the MIC value. Resistance of *M. catarrhalis* to trimethoprim-sulfamethoxazole was still quite unusual and occurred in only 0.5% of the strains. No resistance to amoxacillin-clavulanic acid, the cephalosporins or azithromycin was encountered in this collection of isolates.

The fluoroquinolones, were very active against both *H. influenzae* and *M. catarrhalis* with MIC_{90} values (µg/mL) of 0.03 and 0.06, respectively for both moxifloxacin and levofloxacin. The quinolone MIC values did not vary with beta-lactamase production.

According to the present NCCLS penicillin breakpoints (I: >0.1 – 1.0 µg/mL; R: ≥2.0 µg/mL) of the 5,640 *S. pneumoniae* isolates examined, 64% were fully susceptible, 22% intermediate and 14% were resistant to penicillin.

Dissecting these data more carefully shows that changes in these patterns are influenced by the site of infection, the age of the patient and the geographic location. Among respiratory isolates, 59% were susceptible to penicillin compared to blood isolates in which 72% of the strains were susceptible. So there is a marked difference in the prevalence of resistance depending on the source of the isolate.

Among those patients who are less than 12 years old, the full susceptibility of *S. pneumoniae* to penicillin is lower (58%) and the resistance is concomitantly higher (18%) than in an older population greater than 12 years old (i. e. 66% and 12%). Indeed, among patients that are less than 4 years old, the susceptibility of *S.pneumoniae* to penicillin is only 48%.

There are also geographic differences in terms of the resistance prevalence. Table 1 shows the nine different U.S. Census Bureau regions, which are also used by the Centers for Disease Control and Prevention for tracking other diseases and the nationwide surveillance programs. The East South Central region of the United States had the highest prevalence of resistance to penicillin at 24%. The lowest was in the East North Central United States with 10% resistance. It is clear that there is geographic variability within the United States, underscoring the need for continued surveillance that encompasses a wide geographic berth, patients of different ages and isolates from different sites of infection.

It has been noted that penicillin resistance with *S. pneumoniae* is associated with multiple antibiotic resistance. Table 2 shows the activity of various antimicrobial agents as it pertains to the status of penicillin susceptibility or resis-

Table 1
Geographic distribution
of penicillin resistant
S. pneumoniae in the
United States

Region	No. Sites	% R
New England	14	12%
Mid Atlantic	61	12%
South Atlantic	62	16%
East North Central	82	10%
West North Central	28	15%
East South Central	21	24%
West South Central	31	16%
Montain	19	15%
Pacific	38	12%

Table 2. Associated resistance (% R) among *S. pneumoniae* according to penicillin susceptibility status. Penicillin susceptible (Pen-S), Intermediate (Pen-I), Resistant (Pen-R)

Agent	% R for:		
	Pen S	Pen I	Pen R
Amoxicillin/clav.	0	4.2	60.3
Cefuroxime	0	49.7	99.6
Ceftriaxone	0	2.6	25.8
Erythromycin	6.1	45.5	72.3
Azithromycin	5.3	37.9	64
Trimethoprim-sulfa	5.6	24.5	53.5
Levofloxacin	0	0.2	0.6

tance for *S. pneumoniae*. For every agent that was examined, whether beta-lactam, macrolide or trimethoprim-sulfamethoxazole, the prevalence of resistance correlated with the penicillin resistance. Indeed, a slight increase was seen with levofloxacin as 5 strains were not susceptible.

In contrast, Fig. 1 depicts the moxifloxacin and levofloxacin MIC distributions with the study population of *S. pneumoniae*. The modal MIC value for levofloxacin for over 3,600 strains was 0.5 µg/mL, with that modal distribution being two doubling dilutions from the breakpoint. In comparison, moxifloxacin's modal MIC value was 0.12 µg/mL, 8 times less than the anticipated NCCLS breakpoint of 1.0 µg/mL. It is interesting that the shoulder for MIC distribution

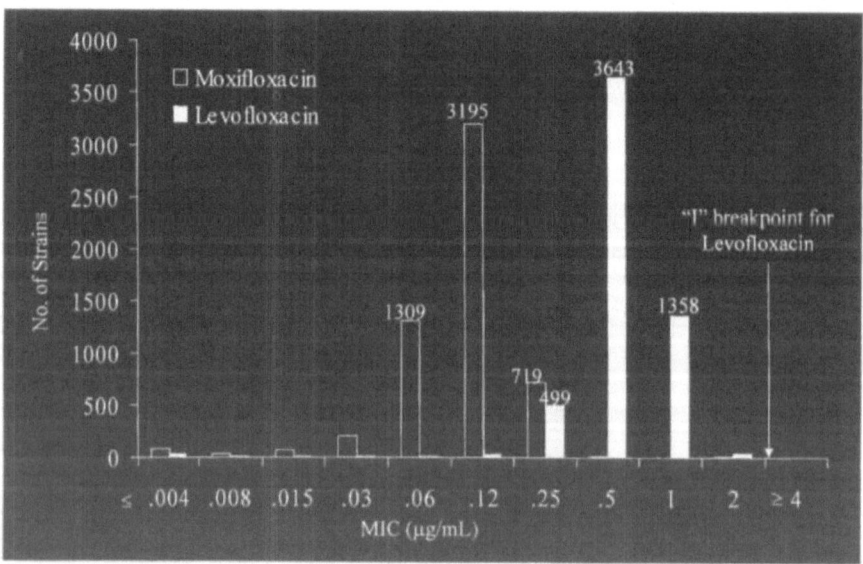

Fig. 1 The distribution of MIC values for moxifloxacin and levofloxacin against pneumococci

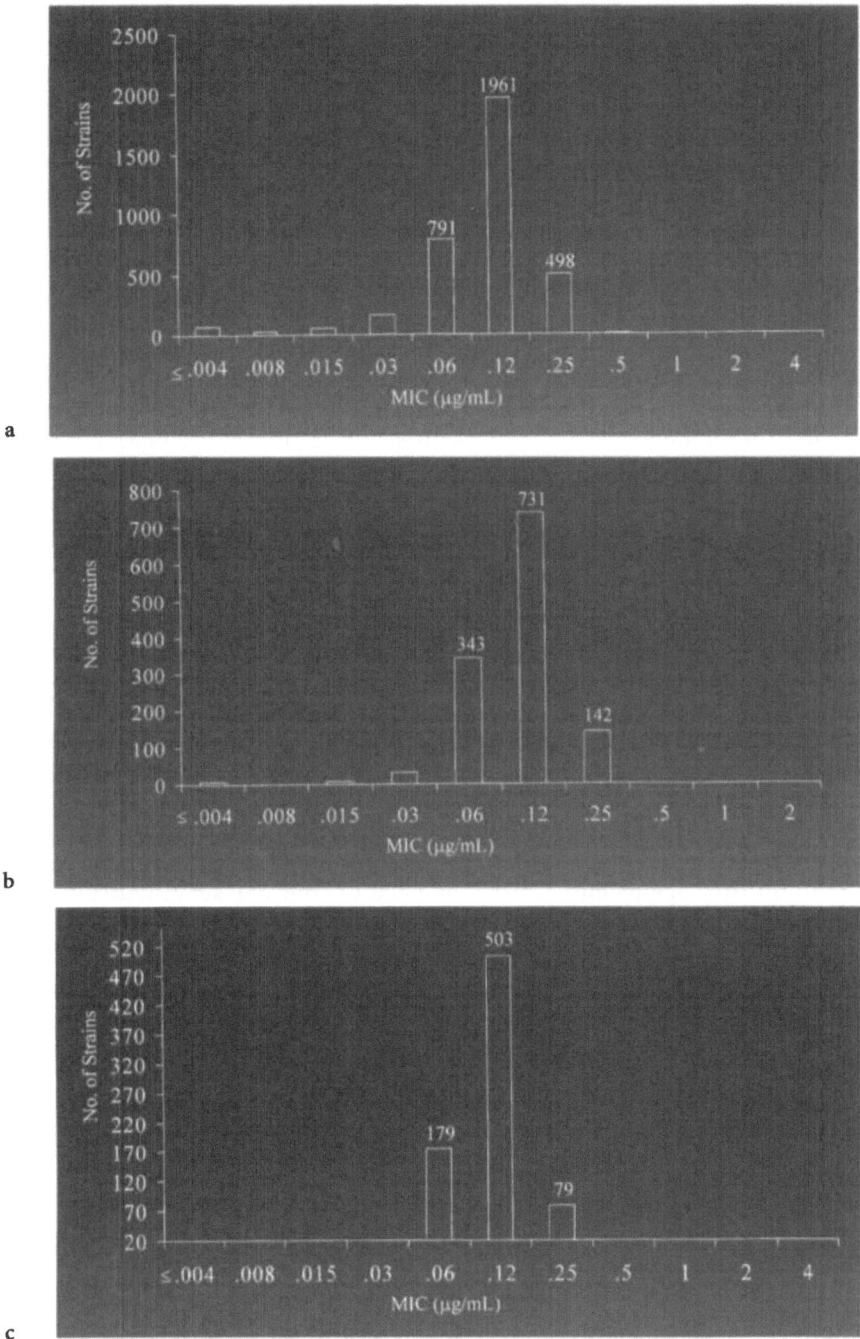

Fig. 2a–c. The distribution of MIC values for moxifloxacin against penicillin susceptible (a), penicillin intermediate (b) and penicillin resistant strains (c) of S. *pneumoniae*

for moxifloxacin showed that the next highest frequency MIC was one dilution below the mode of 0.12 µg/mL. For levofloxacin, the next most frequent MIC value is one dilution higher than the modal MIC value.

Figure 2 depicts the distribution of MIC values for moxifloxacin based on the penicillin status. For penicillin-susceptible strains, (Fig. 2a), the same distribution was found as in Figure 1 with the mode being 0.12 µg/mL and the shoulder at 0.06 µg/mL. With penicillin intermediate strains (Fig. 2b), the distribution was identical with the distribution for the penicillin susceptible strains. There appeared to be no upward shift in the distribution. With the penicillin-resistant population (Fig. 2c), the distribution was exactly the same, the shoulder was at 0.06 µg/mL, the mode at 0.12 µg/mL. These data establish the fact that, currently, the moxifloxacin MIC value distributions are identical regardless of the penicillin status of the isolates. It also underscores the need that, even with very active agents such as moxifloxacin, surveillance has to track MIC value distributions in order to detect what may be subtle, but significant, changes in susceptibility of the organism.

Conclusion

Antimicrobial resistance among *H. influenzae* and *M. catarrhalis* did not appear to be changing in the United States. Penicillin resistance among the pneumococcus was problematic with only 64% of strains isolated being susceptible. Penicillin resistance varied between geographic regions and was most prevalent among respiratory isolates and in younger patients. These factors must be taken into account whenever surveillance studies are conducted. Penicillin resistance was associated with multiple drug resistance with the exception of the fluoroquinolones which continued to maintain a high level of activity, even against multiple-resistant strains. However, the ability of pneumococci to acquire resistance to multiple agents emphasizes the need to continue surveillance of these microorganisms.

CHAPTER 12

Pre-clinical Microbiology – Respiratory Tract Infections Susceptibility Survey – Europe

12

DAVID FELMINGHAM

Abstract. Since 1992, the Alexander Project has monitored the susceptibility of bacterial lower respiratory tract pathogens in Europe, the USA and other parts of the world. In Europe, France and Spain are established as centres of high prevalence penicillin, macrolide and multiple resistance amongst isolates of *Streptococcus pneumoniae*. In other European countries, resistance varies widely according to geographical area. Macrolide resistance is developing both in association with and independently of penicillin resistance, in this species. Beta-lactamase production amongst isolates of *Haemophilus influenzae* is also most prevalent in France and Spain with wide variation between other European centres monitored. Virtually all clinical isolates of *Moraxella catarrhalis* now produce beta-lactamase. Uniquely, resistance to fluoroquinolones occurs infrequently amongst all three species.

Introduction

Respiratory tract infection is a cause of significant morbidity and mortality, worldwide. Most of these infections are viral in origin, however, bacterial species such as *Streptococcus pneumoniae, Haemophilus influenzae* and *Moraxella catarrhalis* are important in community-acquired pneumonia, acute exacerbation of chronic bronchitis, otitis media and sinusitis. Empirical antibacterial therapy for these infections must now take account of the increasing prevalence of resistance phenotypes among the causative organisms which can only be determined by properly conducted susceptibility surveillance studies which, ideally, should be long-term to monitor changes over time. In 1992, supported by an unrestricted educational grant from SmithKline Beecham Pharmaceuticals, Harlow, UK, the Alexander Project was established as a multicentre study of the susceptibility of the three respiratory pathogens detailed above, isolated from patients with community-acquired, lower respiratory tract infection. Originally set up to include centres in the UK, France, Germany, Spain, Italy and the USA, the study was extended in 1996 to include other European centres in the Netherlands, Belgium, Portugal, Switzerland, Austria, Poland, Hungary and the Czech and Slovak Republics [1–5].

Results and Discussion

Streptococcus pneumoniae

Among European countries, France and Spain are established as centres of high prevalence low-level (MIC 0.12-1 µg/mL) and high-level (MIC ≥2 µg/mL) penicillin resistance. Combined low-level and high-level penicillin resistance is also found in excess of 10% of isolates in centres in Hungary, the Slovak Republic, Portugal, Belgium, Switzerland, Poland and the UK, whilst the prevalence of penicillin resistance in Germany, Italy, the Netherlands and Austria is lower (Table 1). Interestingly, from a recent study conducted in Great Britain (England, Wales and Scotland) and Ireland (N. Ireland, UK and Eire), there is a clear difference between the evolution of penicillin resistance in these two geographically distinct areas with high-level resistance observed in excess of 20% of 154 isolates collected from six centres in Ireland compared with 5.6% of 663 isolates from 21 centres in Great Britain [6]. Perhaps of greater interest is the manner in which macrolide resistance is developing in S. pneumoniae. On the one hand, macrolide resistance is strongly associated with penicillin and multiple resistance in this species with centres of high-prevalence in Spain and France (Table 2). However, on closer examination of the susceptibility of isolates from these countries and from Belgium, Switzerland, Germany and Italy, it can be seen that macrolide resistance is also evolving independently of penicillin resistance, in some countries at an alarming rate (e.g. macrolide resistance in Streptococcus pneumoniae occurred in Italy at a prevalence of 1.4% in 1992 rising to 29.8% in 1997) (Table 3).

Resistance to doxycycline, chloramphenicol and, particularly, co-trimoxazole, like macrolide resistance, is also frequently associated with penicillin resistance. However, as with macrolide resistance, resistance to these unrelated antibacterials also occurs independently, presumably reflecting prescription pressure, as is exemplified by the Italian experience, a country where penicillin resistance occurs at low prevalence (Tables 4 and 5). With regard to fluoroquinolone susceptibility, as determined by monitoring the susceptibility of isolates of S. pneumoniae to ciprofloxacin, there has been no change in the mode MIC, MIC_{50} or MIC_{90} after examining a total of 8081 isolates during the period 1992–1997, with less than 1% requiring MIC ≥16 µg/mL (Table 6).

Haemophilus influenzae

The major mechanism of resistance evident amongst isolates of H. influenzae is the production of beta-lactamase which in 1997 was most prevalent in Spain (31.7%), France (19.3%), Belgium (16.1%) and Portugal (12.6%). In the same year, the prevalence of beta-lactamase production in this species was <10% in all other centres, although in both the UK and the Czech Republic it had been higher in previous years. Beta-lactamase negative, ampicillin-resistant (BLNAR) isolates of H. influenzae occurred only rarely, with no clear evolutionary pattern (Table 7).

Table 1. Prevalence of low-level (MIC 0.12-1 µg/mL) and high-level (MIC > 2 µg/mL) penicillin resistance amongst isolates of *Streptococcus pneumoniae*, 1992–1997

Country/centre	Prevalence of penicillin resistance											
	1992		1993		1994		1995		1996		1997	
	low-level	high-level	low-level	high-level	low-level	high-level	low-level	high-level	low-level	high-level	low-level	high-level
France (Paris)	0.1%	0%	13.7%	23.3%	16.7%	31%	20.4%	41.9%	–	–	–	–
France (Toulouse)	20.2%	14.6%	14.5%	21.1%	10.2%	40.1%	14.7%	41.4%	10.3%	32.1%	20.4%	29.3%
Spain (Barcelona)	17.2%	25.1%	17.1%	24.1%	18.6%	30.4%	11.6%	37.8%	18.4%	22.8%	16.6%	34.8%
Spain (Madrid)	–	–	13.5%	40.4%	31.4%	33.3%	14.8%	47.5%	–	–	–	–
UK (London)	0.1%	0.1%	0.2%	0%	0.2%	0%	5.3%	0%	4.5%	4.5%	6.3%	6.3%
UK (Belfast)	0.1%	0%	0.2%	0%	2.4%	11.9%	4.9%	10.8%	–	–	–	–
Italy (Genoa)	14.3%	0%	0%	0%	0.3%	0.2%	9.2%	0.8%	4.2%	4.6%	4.9%	3.1%
Germany (Weingarten)	0.7%	0%	0%	0%	–	–	0.2%	0%	4%	0%	14.5%	0%
The Netherlands									1.5%	3.1%	–	–
Belgium (Leuven)									3.5%	10.1%	4.5%	5.7%
Portugal									–	–	3.5%	16.8%
Switzerland									7.4%	3.2%	5.7%	4.4%
Austria (Vienna)									6.5%	0.9%	–	–
Poland									7.7%	6.4%	5%	9.4%
Hungary									24.4%	11.8%	–	–
The Czech Republic									0%	0%	2.2%	3.2%
The Slovak Republic									3.6%	23.2%	10%	16.7%

NB. Where no particular city/town is indicated, isolates were collected from various centres in the country.

Table 2. Prevalence of macrolide resistance amongst isolates *of Streptococcus pneumoniae,* 1992–1997

Country/centre	Prevalence of macrolide resistance					
	1992	1993	1994	1995	1996	1997
UK (London)	2.3%	4.8%	2.7%	7.4%	13.6%	7.2%
UK (Belfast)	2.6%	0%	0%	3.9%	–	–
France (Paris)	22.5%	50.7%	33.3%	36.6%	–	–
France (Toulouse)	29.2%	27%	46.9%	40.3%	40.6%	45.9%
Spain (Barcelona)	10.1%	11.4%	19.8%	24.4%	19.1%	32.6%
Spain (Madrid)	–	19.2%	52.9%	28.7%	–	–
Germany (Weingarten)	1.7%	0%	12.5%	3.9%	2.7%	6.5%
Italy (Genoa)	1.4%	5.2%	14.8%	20.8%	24.1%	29.8%
The Netherlands					1.5%	–
Belgium (Leuven)					22%	31.1%
Portugal					–	3.5%
Switzerland					6.4%	15.8%
Austria (Vienna)					4.6%	–
Poland					12.2%	13.7%
Hungary					13.4%	–
The Czech Republic					0%	2.2%
The Slovak Republic					17.9%	13.3%

NB. Where no particular city/town is indicated, isolates were collected from various centres in the country.

Table 3. Prevalence of macrolide resistance amongst isolates *of Streptococcus pneumoniae –* relationship between penicillin and macrolide susceptibility (1997 isolates)

Country/centre	Prevalence of macrolide resistance amongst isolates exhibiting		
	Penicillin susceptibility	Penicillin low-level resistance	Penicillin high-level resistance
France (Toulouse)	13.2%	75.7%	81.1%
Belgium (Leuven)	29.5%	33.3%	53.3%
Spain (Barcelona)	7.1%	65.5%	52.5%
Switzerland	13.4%	11%	60%
Germany (Weingarten)	7.5%	0%	–
Italy (Genoa)	21.3%	70%	36.4%

NB. Where no particular city/town is indicated, isolates were collected from various centres in the country.

Table 4. Doxycycline, chloramphenicol and co-trimoxazole resistance amongst isolates of *Streptococcus pneumoniae*, 1997

High prevalence doxycycline resistance (%)
    France, Toulouse = 25.4, Spain, Barcelona = 39.4, Belgium, Leuven = 25.4,
    Italy, Genoa = 27.2, the Slovak Republic = 15, Poland = 40.3

High prevalence chloramphenicol resistance (%)
    France, Toulouse = 14.9, Spain, Barcelona = 33.7, Italy, Genoa = 16.2,
    the Slovak Republic = 16.7, Poland = 15.8

High prevalence co-trimoxazole resistace (%)
    France, Toulouse = 38.7, Spain, Barcelona = 60.6, Belgium, Leuven = 24.2,
    Portugal = 23.9, Italy, Genoa = 37.7, the Slovak Republic = 25, Hungary = 55.1,
    Poland = 35.3

Table 5. Doxycycline, chloramphenicol and co-trimoxazole resistance amongst isolates of *Streptococcus pneumoniae* from Genoa, Italy, 1992–1997

Antibiotic	Prevalence of resistance					
	1992	1993	1994	1995	1996	1997
Doxycycline	12.9	5.2	20.3	18.5	22.8	27.2
Chloramphenicol	14.3	17.2	5.5	13.8	7.6	16.2
Co-trimoxazole	30	20.7	35.2	36.2	35.9	37.7

Table 6. Ciprofloxacin susceptibility of isolates of *Streptococcus pneumoniae*, 1992–1997

Activity	Ciprofloxacin susceptibility					
	1992 (903)	1993 (953)	1994 (973)	1995 (1056)	1996 (2160)	1997 (2036)
Mode MIC µg/mL	1	0,5	1	1	1	1
MIC$_{50}$ µg/mL	1	0,5	1	1	1	1
MIC$_{90}$ µg/mL	2	1	2	2	2	2

The activity of the macrolides, against isolates of *H. influenzae* has followed an essentially unimodal distribution in the rank order of potency; azithromycin (mode MIC 0.5-1 µg/mL) > erythromycin (mode MIC 4 µg/mL) > clarithromycin (mode MIC 4-8 µg/mL), throughout the period 1992–1997 with no evidence of the development of resistance. The fluoroquinolones, ciprofloxacin (MIC$_{90}$ 0.03 µg/mL) and ofloxacin (MIC$_{90}$ 0.12 µg/mL) have remained potently active against *H. influenzae* with only 12/11,539 strains (0.1%) examined between 1992–1997 exhibiting resistance (Table 8).

Table 7. Prevalence of beta-lactamase production and beta-lactamase negative, ampicillin resistance (BLNAR) amongst isolates of *Haemophilus influenzae*, 1992–1997

Country/centre	Prevalence of beta-lactamase production and BLNAR	1992	1993	1994	1995	1996	1997
UK (London)	β-lactamase production	6.5%	10.9%	6.9%	16.7%	14.2%	6.3%
	BLNAR	–	–	0.5%	0%	0%	0%
UK (Belfast)	β-lactamase production	7%	13.9%	18.4%	12.8%	–	–
	BLNAR	–	–	0%	0.7%	–	–
France (Paris)	β-lactamase production	–	18.5%	20.3%	25.5%	–	–
	BLNAR	–	–	0%	0%	–	–
France (Toulouse)	β-lactamase production	16.7%	20.9%	18.7%	17.2%	19.8%	19.3%
	BLNAR	–	–	0.5%	0.6%	0%	0%
Spain (Barcelona)	β-lactamase production	38.5%	23.5%	25%	26%	26%	31.7%
	BLNAR	–	–	1%	2%	1.8%	0%
Spain (Madrid)	β-lactamase production	31.9%	34.2%	24.7%	25%	–	–
	BLNAR	–	–	0.6%	0%	–	–
Italy (Genoa)	β-lactamase production	3.8%	6.3%	11.2%	4%	1.8%	2%
	BLNAR	–	–	0%	0%	0%	0%
Germany (Weingarten)	β-lactamase production	5.6%	1.4%	3%	13.1%	5%	6%
	BLNAR	–	–	0%	0%	0%	0%
the Netherlands	β-lactamase production					4.1%	–
	BLNAR					0%	–
Belgium (Leuven)	β-lactamase production					21.9%	16.1%
	BLNAR					0%	0%
Portugal	β-lactamase production					–	12.6%
	BLNAR					–	0.5%
Switzerland	β-lactamase production					8.1%	7.1%
	BLNAR					0%	0%
Austria (Vienna)	β-lactamase production					5.2%	–
	BLNAR					0%	–
Poland	β-lactamase production					3.8%	5.6%
	BLNAR					0%	0%
Hungary	β-lactamase production					0%	–
	BLNAR					0%	–
The Czech Republic	β-lactamase production					13%	7.9%
	BLNAR					0%	0%
The Slovak Republic	β-lactamase production					4.8%	5.3%
	BLNAR					0%	2.6%

BLNAR = β-lactamase negative, ampicillin resistant (MIC ≥4 mg/L).

Table 8. In-vitro activity of macrolides and fluoroquinolones against isolates of *Haemophilus influenzae* and *Moraxella catarrhalis*

	In vitro activity	
	Haemophilus influenzae	*Moraxella catarrhalis*
Macrolides	mode MIC (μg/mL)	mode MIC (μg/mL)
Erythromycin	4	0.12
Clarithromycin	4 – 8	0.06
Azithromycin	0.5 – 1	0.03
	[no changes during surveillance period]	[no changes during surveillance period]
Fluoroquinolones	MIC$_{90}$ (μg/mL)	MIC$_{90}$ (μg/mL)
Ciprofloxacin	0.03	0.06
Ofloxacin	0.12	0.12
	[13/11,539 (0.1%) fluoroquinolone resistant]	[1/2,998 (0.03%) fluoroquinolone resistant]

Moraxella catarrhalis

The only mechanism of resistance of any importance encountered in this species is the production of beta-lactamase with more than 90% of isolates examined doing so. All clinical isolates of *M. catarrhalis* must now be considered resistant to penicillin and the amino-penicillins (except these combined with an inhibitor of beta-lactamase). As with *H. influenzae*, the fluoroquinolones, ciprofloxacin (MIC$_{90}$ 0.06 μg/mL) and ofloxacin (MIC$_{90}$ 0.12 μg/mL), have remained highly active against *M. catarrhalis* throughout the period of study with only 1 strain (0.03%) out of 2998 isolates tested apparently fluoroquinolone-resistant (Table 8).

Conclusions

Empirical therapy of respiratory tract infection must take account of the increasing prevalence of antimicrobial resistance amongst the three principal bacterial pathogens, *S. pneumoniae*, *H. influenzae* and *M. catarrhalis*. Penicillin, macrolide and multiple resistance are the main concerns amongst isolates of *S. pneumoniae* with considerable variation in their prevalence between European countries whilst amongst isolates of *H. influenzae*, beta-lactamase production is the principal mechanism of resistance. Clinical isolates of *M. catarrhalis* must now be considered inherent producers of beta-lactamase. Geographically, antimicrobial resistance is generally more prevalent in Mediterranean and Eastern European countries than in other areas. Uniquely, fluoroquinolone resistance is observed only rarely in all three species. However, the only moderate activity of ciprofloxacin and ofloxacin against *S. pneumoniae* is of concern. New fluoroquinolones with improved potency against *S. pneumoniae* and retained activity against *H. influenzae* and *M. catarrhalis*, such as moxifloxacin [7], offer new treatment opportunities for bacterial respiratory tract infections.

References

1. Felmingham D, Grüneberg RN, Alexander Project Group (1996) A multicentre, collaborative study of the antimicrobial susceptibility of community-acquired, lower respiratory tract pathogens 1992–1993: the Alexander Project Journal of Antimicrobial Chemotherapy 38 Suppl A : 11–57
2. Felmingham D, Washington J, Alexander Project Group (1999) Trends in the antimicrobial susceptibility of bacterial respiratory tract pathogens – findings of the Alexander Project 1992–1996. Journal of Chemotherapy 11, Suppl 1:5–21
3. Felmingham D, Grüneberg RN, Alexander Project Group (1998) The Alexander Project 1996–1997: a continuing, international, multicentre study of the antimicrobial susceptibility of community-acquired lower respiratory tract bacterial pathogens – *Moraxella catarrhalis.* Abstracts of the 2nd European Congress of Chemotherapy, Hamburg, Germany. Poster T246
4. Felmingham D, Grüneberg RN, Alexander Project Group (1998) The Alexander Project 1996–1997: a continuing, international, multicentre study of the antimicrobial susceptibility of community-acquired lower respiratory tract bacterial pathogens – *Haemophilus influenzae.* Abstracts of the 2nd European Congress of Chemotherapy, Hamburg, Germany. Poster T247
5. Felmingham D, Grüneberg RN, Alexander Project Group (1999) The Alexander Project 1996–1997: a continuing, international, multicentre study of the antimicrobial susceptibility of community-acquired lower respiratory tract bacterial pathogens – *Streptococcus pneumoniae.* Abstracts of the 2nd European Congress of Chemotherapy, Hamburg, Germany. Poster T248
6. Masterton RG, Felmingham D, Burley C (1998) A UK, multicentre study of the antimicrobial susceptibility of clinical respiratory tract isolates of *Streptococcus pneumoniae* cultured from patients with lower respiratory tract infection during the 1997–1998 cold season. Programme and Abstracts of the 6th International Symposium on New Quinolones, Denver, Colorado, USA, p 48
7. Blondeau J (1999) A review of the comparative in vitro activities of 12 antimicrobial agents, with a focus on five new "respiratory quinolones". Journal of Antimicrobial Chemotherapy, 43, Suppl B, 1–11

Pre-clinical Microbiology – Respiratory Tract Infections Susceptibility Survey – Japan

Kazunori Tomono

Abstract. *Streptococcus pneumoniae, Haemophilus influenzae* and *Moraxella catarrhalis* are major aetiologic agents of respiratory tract infections in Japan as in other countries. Recently, penicillin-resistant *S. pneumoniae* (PRSP) have been isolated all over the world, concurrently prevalence of these strains has increased dramatically in Japan. In 1998, four clinical isolates of high-level resistance to fluoroquinolones, including sparfloxacin, were found in Okinawa prefecture, the southern islands of Japan. *S. pneumoniae*, which shows high-level resistance to fluoroquinolones, may be a problem organism in the future unless appropriate dosing is followed. The prevalence of beta-lactamase producing *H. influenzae* has not increased recently. All of *M. catarrhalis* isolated in 1996 and 1997 at Nagasaki University Hospital produced beta-lactamase.

Introduction

There is a risk of a rapid increase in infectious diseases in Japan and with it the serious problem of drug resistant pathogens. Penicillin-resistant *Streptococcus pneumoniae* (PRSP) and methicillin-resistant *Staphylococcus aureus* (MRSA) are the major problem organisms in community clinics as well as in hospitals. This presentation will review the results of national Japanese surveys of respiratory tract pathogens.

Results and Discussion

In Japan, as in other countries, *S. pneumoniae, Haemophilus influenzae* and *Moraxella catarrhalis* are major respiratory tract pathogens. A recent Japanese survey of over 300 patients with community acquired pneumonia (CAP) who required hospitalization showed *S. pneumoniae* was the most common pathogen with an incidence of 23%. This was followed by *H. influenzae* at 7.4%, *Mycoplasma pneumoniae* at 4.9% and *Klebsiella pneumoniae* at 4.3%. The incidence of *M. catarrhalis* was 1.8% [1].

There are changes evident in the pathogens isolated from the sputum of pneumonia patients. The data in Figure 1 shows the frequency of pathogens isolated from the sputum at university hospital in Nagasaki. These profiles are not specific to one hospital, but are similar throughout Japan. The frequency of *H. influenzae* decreased during the 1980's due to the introduction of treatment with quinolones. *Pseudomonas aeruginosa* has been consistently found in

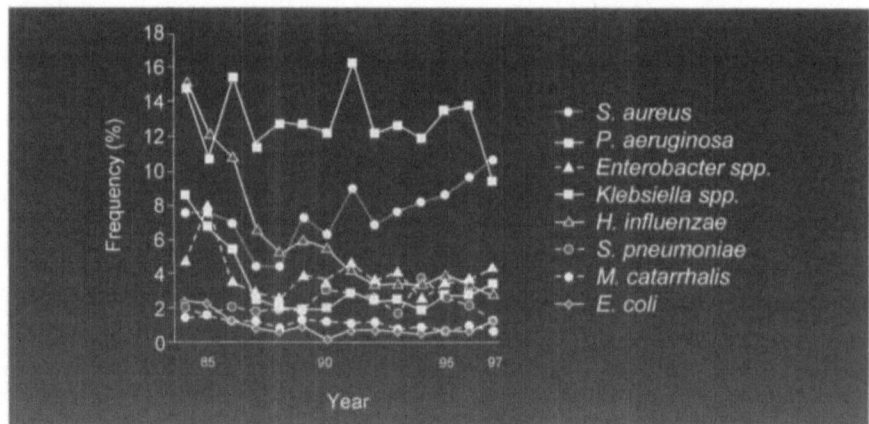

Fig. 1. Annual changes in bacterial isolates from sputum patients at University Hospital in Nagasaki, Japan

sputum from patients at most university hospitals. The increase in *S. aureus* was probably due to the epidemic of MRSA among patients with respiratory infections.

Broad spectrum antibiotics have been prescribed for community respiratory tract infections as well as for critical cases in hospitals. This may have been responsible for the rapid increase and high frequency of beta-lactamase resistant bacteria in Japan. This phenomenon may be closely related to the health care system in Japan, where health insurance is widespread, and permits Japanese physicians to prescribe any antibiotic provided it has been approved for treating pneumonia. Thus, empirical therapy with parenteral agents may involve an iv infusion for a young patient suspected of having CAP, without there being any identification of the infecting organism or of any underlying complication. Penicillin may be a viable option in this type of uncomplicated patient until a causative agent is identified.

The prevalence of PRSP in Asian countries (Fig. 2) was derived from the Asian Network for Surveillance of Resistant Pneumococci (ANSORP). The highest prevalences of PRSP were found in Korea, Japan and Thailand; in contrast, there was a low prevalence in India and China. Lately, new generation fluoroquinolones have been developed with high antimicrobial activity against pneumococci, including PRSP. They will probably become first line drugs to treat CAP. However, it was recently reported that four clinical isolates of *S. pneumoniae* were highly resistant to ciprofloxacin and sparfloxacin (see Table 1).

The distribution of MIC values for 150 clinical isolates of *S. pneumoniae* was determined for sparfloxacin [2]; MIC_{90} values were 2.0 and 0.5 μg/mL, respectively. The distribution of MIC values (Fig. 3) shows that there were a small number of isolates with a MIC value above 16.

The clinical profile of 4 patients from whom quinolone-resistant *S. pneumoniae* were isolated is shown in Table 1. Three of those patients had been treated with sparfloxacin, levofloxacin or CS-940, a new fluoroquinolone developed in

Fig. 2
The prevalence of penicillin-resistant
S. pneumoniae in Asian countries. The data
were taken from the Asian Network for
Surveillance of resistant pneumococci
(ANSORP), May 1996 – April 1997

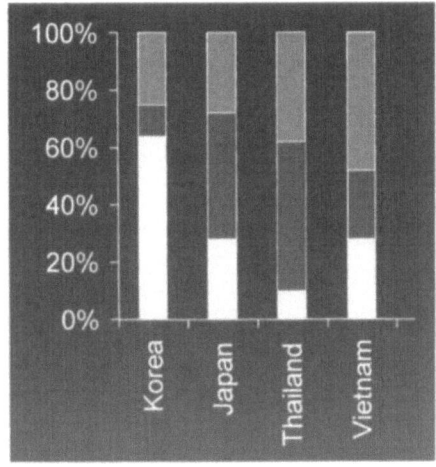

Fig. 3
The distribution of MIC
values [2] for ciprofloxacin
and sparfloxacin against
150 clinical isolates of
S. pneumoniae

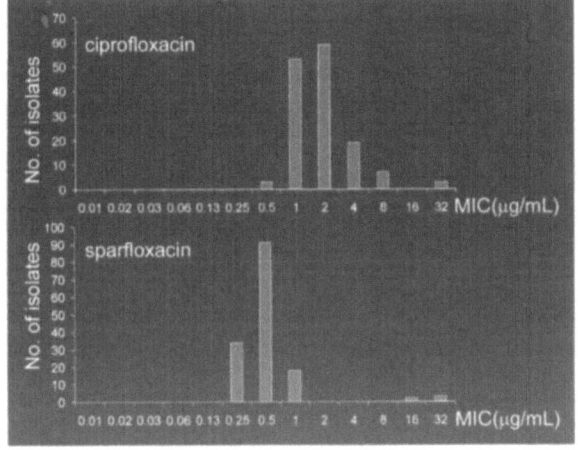

Japan. One highly resistant strain (252) was isolated from the patient's blood during treatment with clindamycin and vancomycin. When compared against a fluoroquinolone-susceptible strain, each of the resistant strains showed mutations in both the *GyrA* regions and the *ParC* regions; this was especially so for strain 252, one of the highly resistant strains. So, although the new generation of fluoroquinolones, like trovafloxacin and moxifloxacin, have potentially useful activity against pneumococci and may become the first choice for treating CAP, it will be important to pay attention to the emergence of resistant strains due to extensive use of other less effective quinolones which could lead to a serious problem such as PRSP.

The surveys have shown that 10–20% of *H. influenzae* in Japanese hospitals are beta-lactamase producers. The prevalence was highest at 20–25% around 1990. This decrease may have occurred due to the increased use of cephems,

Table 1. The profiles [2] of four clinical isolates of sparfloxacin resistant *S. pneumoniae*. All strains were of serotype 23

Strain	Relevant characteristics	MIC (µg/mL)		
		PCG	CPFX	SPFX
182	Isolate from sputum of a 76 yr old male patient treated with sparfloxacin and levofloxacin	1.0	64	16
674	Isolate from sputum of a 74 yr old male patient during CS-940 treatment	0.25	64	64
354	Isolate from sputum of a 74 yr old male patient after CS-940 treatment	0.25	64	128
252	Isolate from blood of a 33 yr old male patient treated with ampicillin, imipenem-cilastatin, clindamycin and vancomycin	0.25	64	128

PCG – penicillin G; CPFX – ciprofloxacin; SPFX – sparfloxacin and CS-940 a new fluoroquinolone developed in Japan (MIC 8 µg/mL). The MIC for levofloxacin was 16 µg/mL.

Table 2. The activity of fluoroquinolones against respiratory pathogens

Organism	Test Drug	No of Isolates	MIC value (µg/mL)		
			Range	MIC_{50}	MIC_{90}
PSSP	Moxi	30	0.05–0.20	0.20	0.20
	Cipro	30	0.20–0.78	0.78	0.78
	Levo	30	0.20–0.78	0.78	0.78
PRSP	Moxi	30	0.10–1.56	0.20	0.20
+	Cipro	30	0.39–12.5	0.78	1.56
PISP	Levo	30	0.20–6.25	0.78	0.78
H.influenzae	Moxi	30	≤0.025–0.05	≤0.025	0.05
	Cipro	30	≤0.025–0.05	≤0.025	≤0.025
	Levo	30	≤0.025–0.05	≤0.025	≤0.05
M.catarrhalis	Moxi	30	≤0.025–0.05	≤0.05	≤0.05
	Cipro	30	≤0.025–0.05	≤0.05	≤0.05
	Levo	30	≤0.025–0.10	≤0.05	≤0.10

PSSP – penicillin susceptible *S. pneumoniae* with MIC_{90} of < 0.06 µg/mL.
PRSP – penicillin resistant *S. pneumoniae* with MIC_{90} of > 2 µg/mL.
PISP – penicillin intermediate *S. pneumoniae* with MIC_{90} of 0.12 – 1 µg/mL.

carbapenems and fluoroquinolones to which *H. influenzae* are very sensitive. *M. catarrhalis* is frequently isolated from respiratory tract infections, mainly from acute exacerbations of chronic bronchitis. Almost all the clinical isolates of *M. catarrhalis* show beta-lactamase activity, although this is not a major concern because there is little evidence of resistance to macrolides or fluoroquinolones.

The results in Table 2 show the latest data of the antibacterial activity of moxifloxacin against clinical isolates from patients with respiratory tract infections in Japan. The MIC_{90} values for moxifloxacin were 0.20 µg/mL against both penicillin-susceptible and penicillin-resistant strains of *S. pneumoniae*. The activity against *H. influenzae* and *M. catarrhalis* was equivalent to ciprofloxacin and levofloxacin. Clearly, moxifloxacin exhibits potent activity against respiratory pathogens, including PRSP. It will become one of the first line drugs to treat mild to moderate CAP without complications. Careful monitoring will be necessary to prevent an epidemic of fluoroquinolone-resistant strains, especially of pneumococcus.

References

1. Ishida T, Hashimoto T, Arita M, Ito I, Osawa M (1998) Etiology of community acquired pneumonia in hospitalized patients – a 3 year prospective study in Japan. Chest 114 (6): 1588–1593
2. Taba H, Kusano N (1998) Sparfloxacin resistance in clinical isolates of Streptococcus pneumoniae: Involvement of multiple mutations in Gyr A and Par C genes. Antimicrobial Agents and Chemotherapy 42 (9): 2193–2196

Discussion on Respiratory Tract Infections Susceptibility Surveys

QUESTION: One of the interesting things is how you look at pneumococcal isolates from blood and lung tissue and show differences. In one of our studies, and in looking at data from other investigators, there is a suggestion that there are differences in the susceptibilities of *H. influenzae*, depending whether they are respiratory or sinus isolates. Do you have any information on that?

ANSWER: We do, but we did not include them in the presentation. It seems as though the only difference would be in beta-lactamase production since there is not a lot of resistance to other drugs except trimethoprim sulpha. Beta-lactamase production was much higher, as one would expect, in sinus infections which are frequently undertreated, mistreated and not treated long enough. This may lead to the development of resistance in multiple bacterial isolates.

QUESTION: I understand. The other problem that we encounter in doing our surveillance is the true paucity of systemic *H. influenzae* infections in blood or spinal fluid in the United States.

1st ANSWER: I would comment that we have similar experience in our isolates from sinuses. That is, there are higher rates of beta-lactamase producing strains.

Our explanation is that the sinus is a much more compartmentalised habitat in comparison with the throat and so the competition between different populations of bacteria is much less frequent. Therefore, if you do not eradicate the bacteria in the sinus, the resistant ones will prevail. These resistant populations may be killed just by competition in the throat.

2nd ANSWER: I recall two clinical studies which we did in the United Kingdom, one with ciprofloxacin and one with Augmentin. We looked at patients with so-called acute bronchitis and those with acute exacerbations of chronic bronchitis. There was a difference in the beta-lactamase prevalence amongst the isolates of *H. influenzae*. The prevalence was twice as high in those patients who had acute exacerbations of chronic bronchitis compared to those who had apparent acute bronchitis.

QUESTION: I have a question about the emergence of macrolide resistance in *S. pneumoniae*. Some studies have suggested that the mechanism in Europe may be more ERM-based whereas in the United States it is more an efflux mechanism. Based on all these surveillance studies that have been presented, do we have enough evidence to conclude that there are continental differences in the macrolide resistance mechanisms of *S. pneumoniae* and, if so, what is the explanation for it?

1st ANSWER: We have data based on using macrolide and clindamycin phenotypes to mark the M-type of resistance. In the United States now, the breakdown is approximately 67 % which appear to have the efflux phenotype and the remainder are ERM-based which is typical of the European strains with high level resistance to clindamycin and the macrolides. I have no explanation for the difference between continents, but I would be glad to entertain any thoughts that my colleague may have.

2nd ANSWER: We have the opposite. We have about 15 to 20 % of the M-phenotype and efflux mechanism. The remainder in Europe is ERM-based. By the way, some strains that appear at first view to have the efflux phenotype may in fact have the ERM mechanism. It is not the typical marker that counts, it should be compared to biogenetically characterised organisms.

3rd ANSWER: From the point of view of our study, we recognise this is now a very interesting issue and that it also includes clindamycin. It will be interesting to go back and look at some of the isolates which are still retained from previous years. So, no data at the moment, but the problem is recognised.

QUESTION: Your studies have looked at macrolides, I think azithromycin, whereas others have looked at clarithromycin. One of the big problems in the U.S. is clarithromycin resistance in *H. influenzae* and clinical failures. Do you have any feeling for the difference in sensitivity of *H. influenzae* to the macrolides and how bad it is getting for certain macrolides?

1st ANSWER: I did not include the clarithromycin data in the presentation, but it is basically the same as Dr. Felmingham has alluded to. It is not so much the category of resistance, it is the natural MIC distribution of *H. influenzae* to clarithromycin. Their MIC_{50} and MIC_{90} values would be higher to clarithromycin than to azithromycin. It is closely connected to the biology of the organism and I do not know whether there is emerging resistance or that is the level of resistance that this organism has always had.

2nd ANSWER: The distribution curves suggest that there is no true mechanism of macrolide resistance in *H. influenzae* probably because these agents have been so weakly active that the selection pressure has not been expressed on *H. influenzae* populations. Obviously with better macrolides, eventually we may see something. It looks like there is a shift to higher level resistance in *H. influenzae*, at least to clarithromycin, than there was five years ago. Is this true? It appears that it`s coming out of the TRUST studies which have shown that there is more clarithromycin resistance than was seen in the past.

3rd ANSWER: The problem is using arbitrary breakpoints to define susceptibility and resistance to the macrolides. They do not tell you anything microbiologically, because there is a normal distribution, a unimodel distribution, for all three macrolides. To my understanding, there are inadequate clinical data to support the use of some defining breakpoint to separate one of three compounds all of which have relatively poor activity against *H. influenzae*. I do not think resistance is changing from the data that we have on 12,000 isolates and neither has the modal distribution changed. So it appears that since 1990, with a large number of organisms, there is no change in the susceptibility of *H. influenzae* to the macrolides.

With regard to the previous observation about differences in susceptibility rates depending on respiratory or blood isolates or isolates obtained from the sinus, one of the points you emphasize is that you wanted to have good denominators. When we report resistance data based solely on whole populations in these networks, it does not really help clinicians because I would suspect that there are tremendous confounders. For example, trivial isolates obtained from ear infections in well-appearing children are much different than deep respiratory isolates from ICU patients with CAP. I suspect that blood is obtained from sicker patients and so that data may be more important. Those patients who come to get maxillary aspirates of their sinusitis are much different, probably have been exposed to therapies for a more prolonged amount of time, but might represent a minority of patients that I treat for common acute sinusitis. So, to the extent that all these networks can stratify their data and analyse these groups separately, I think the information would be much more meaningful to us who try to use the data clinically.

4th ANSWER: I think you are right. We still do have a need for more clear-cut epidemiology at different locations. We need the worldwide data, we need nationwide data and so on.

QUESTION: One of the major pressures to use moxifloxacin is going to be if we find that there are clinical failures for PRSP treated with penicillins. The only evidence so far that that is going to happen is with patients who have infections due to organisms with MIC values of 2 µg/mL or above. I was wondering if our colleagues could tell us from all these surveys, what proportion of these organisms are actually present in these surveillance studies?

1st ANSWER: Obviously, that varies from country to country. The number of strains having MIC values over 2 µg/mL is still increasing in Spain and in France. There is about 20% incidence in Barcelona of organisms with a MIC value of 2 µg/mL for penicillin. Fortunately, there are no strains with MIC values greater than 4 µg/mL, though that may happen in the future. It is possible to do gene transfer into *S. pneumoniae* and obtain strains with MIC values in excess of 100 µg/mL.

2nd ANSWER: In our surveillance, we had 10 strains that had MIC values greater than 8 µg/mL to penicillin. To the point about clinical relevance of some of the surveillance, I think that there are reasons to do it, not only for the sake of the patient, but for the sake of tracking what the microbiological population is doing. There is no doubt, whether or not it is clinically relevant, that the pneumococci we are seeing today are completely different than the pneumococci that we saw 15 years ago.

CHAPTER 14

Mechanisms of Fluoroquinolone Action and Resistance

14

KARL DRLICA

Abstract. Intracellular fluoroquinolone action involves two steps. First, drug-topoisomerase-DNA complexes form in which the DNA is broken. These complexes reversibly block DNA replication and bacterial growth. Second, lethal DNA breaks are released from the complexes. Inhibitors of protein synthesis, such as chloramphenicol, block cell death and the release of DNA breaks from complexes trapped by oxolinic acid, a first generation quinolone. However, they only partially protect cells from the lethal action of fluoroquinolones, suggesting that these compounds act by the chloramphenicol-sensitive pathway and by a second pathway. Resistance to fluoroquinolones arises step-wise from mutations in the two intracellular targets, DNA gyrase and DNA topoisomerase IV. Addition of a methoxy group to N1-cyclopropyl fluoroquinolones improves bacteriostatic and bactericidal action, especially against first-step, resistant mutants. Consequently, C-8-methoxy derivatives restrict the selection of resistance by bacterial populations, a feature that has been shown for several bacterial species including clinical MDR isolates of *Mycobacterium tuberculosis*. Since minimum inhibitory concentration (MIC) against wild-type cells fails to accurately predict attack of resistant mutants or selection of resistance, a new parameter called mutant prevention concentration (MPC) is proposed as an additional measure of quinolone potency.

The chromosome of *Escherichia coli* is composed of a single, double-stranded DNA circle that is more than 1,000 μm long. To fit within a bacterial cell that is only 1 to 3 μm long, chromosomal DNA must undergo tertiary folding and compaction. One level of compaction may arise from macromolecular crowding created by the high concentration of solutes in the cytoplasm. Another probably involves long-range folding through the arrangement of DNA into 50 to 80 topologically independent domains. A third level derives from the negative supercoils present in chromosomal DNA, and a fourth must come from the presence of small DNA bending proteins. Within this context the DNA is synthesized at a rate of 50,000 bp per minute per replication fork. For replication to occur efficiently, the DNA strands must readily separate. Moreover, tangles, crossovers (precatenates), and catenates (intermolecular interlinks) must be quickly removed. These and other topological problems are solved by enzymes called DNA topoisomerases. Two of these enzymes, DNA gyrase and DNA topoisomerase IV are targets of the fluoroquinolones (reviewed in [1]).

Gyrase, which is encoded by the *gyrA* and *gyrB* genes, is responsible for introducing negative supercoils into DNA and for relieving topological stress arising from the translocation of transcription and replication complexes along DNA. The enzyme acts by wrapping DNA into a positive supercoil and then passing one region of duplex DNA through another via DNA breakage and rejoining.

Topoisomerase IV is a homologue of gyrase that is encoded by the *parC* and *parE* genes. Its reaction mechanism is similar to that of gyrase, but topoisomerase IV binds to DNA crossovers rather than wrapping DNA. Topoisomerase IV is involved primarily with the unlinking of replicated daughter chromosomes, a process that is called decatenation.

The fluoroquinolones act by binding to complexes that form between DNA and gyrase or topoisomerase IV. Shortly after binding, the quinolones induce a conformational change in the enzyme. The enzymes break DNA, and the quinolones prevent re-ligation of the broken DNA strands, thereby trapping the topoisomerases on DNA as ternary drug-enzyme-DNA complexes. Complex formation reversibly blocks DNA synthesis, and so it is generally thought to be responsible for the bacteriostatic action of the quinolones. We use minimum inhibitory concentration (MIC) as a physiological indicator of complex formation.

The consequences of ternary complex formation differ for the two enzymes, probably because they occur at different places on the chromosome. For example, attack of gyrase by the quinolones inhibits DNA replication rapidly, consistent with gyrase acting ahead of replication forks. In contrast, inhibition of replication by topoisomerase IV-mediated complexes occurs slowly, consistent with this enzyme being located behind replication forks. Indeed, quinolone attack of topoisomerase IV can occur on plasmid DNA without affecting DNA synthesis [2].

Lethal action, at least when gyrase is the quinolone target, is a separate event from complex formation: higher concentrations are required to kill cells than to block growth or form ternary complexes. Moreover, some quinolones block growth better than others but are less effective at killing cells [3]. One hint about the mechanism of lethal action comes from the observation that cell death caused by older quinolones, such as oxolinic acid, is blocked by inhibitors of protein synthesis even though inhibition of replication, and presumably complex formation, is not. Apparently a suicide protein is induced that is responsible for cell death. Little is known about this putative protein factor.

Our working hypothesis is that cell death arises from the release of DNA ends from quinolone-gyrase-DNA complexes (Fig. 1). Support for this idea emerged from sedimentation analysis of isolated bacterial nucleoids [4]. When sedimented into a series of sucrose density-gradients containing increasing concentrations of ethidium bromide, the nucleoid sedimentation coefficient decreases as negative supercoils are removed by the dye until a minimum sedimentation rate is observed. At higher ethidium concentrations positive supercoils are introduced, and the sedimentation coefficient increases. If breaks are introduced into the DNA by treatment with DNase, the supercoils relax and ethidium bromide has little effect on the sedimentation coefficient. Treatment of cells with lethal concentrations of oxolinic acid also flattens the response of nucleoid sedimentation rate to ethidium bromide. Chloramphenicol, an inhibitor of protein synthesis that blocks the lethal activity of oxolinic acid, prevents the flattening of the ethidium-sedimentation rate curve.

With fluoroquinolones such as ciprofloxacin, chloramphenicol only partially blocks lethal action, and it has little effect on the ability of fluoroquinolones to flatten ethidium titration curves when the sedimentation of isolated nucleoids is measured [4]. Thus there must be two lethal modes of quinolone action, one that

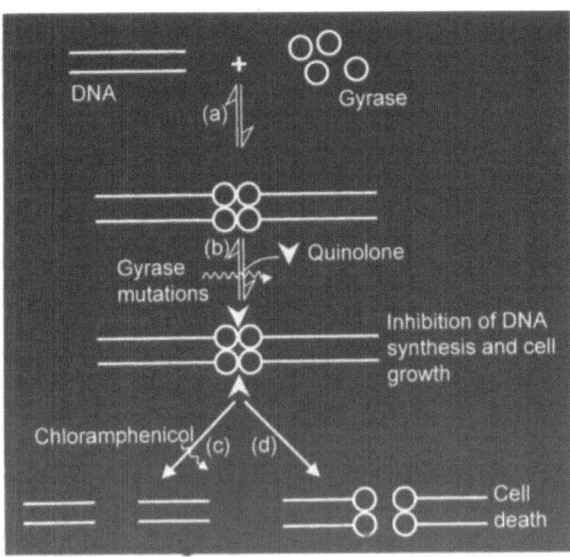

Fig. 1. Intracellular action of fluoroquinolones. (a) DNA plus gyrase or topoisomerase IV form a complex with DNA. (b) Quinolones bind to the complex, altering the conformation of the protein, enhancing a distortion in the DNA, and preventing religation after the protein cleaves DNA. This traps the topoisomerase on DNA in such a way that DNA replication and cell growth are blocked. Trapping topoisomerases on DNA is reversible; consequently, trapping is considered to be bacteriostatic. (c) One form of lethal action occurs by a protein-dependent release of DNA breaks from the complexes, since chloramphenicol blocks the release of breaks and the lethal action of some quinolones. (d) A second pathway to cell death is insensitive to chloramphenicol and is depicted as arising from dissociation of the topoisomerase subunits

requires protein synthesis and one that does not. We have suggested that the chloramphenicol-insensitive mode arises from the stimulation of gyrase subunit dissociation [4].

Many clinically important bacterial species are sensitive to fluoroquinolones such as ciprofloxacin and levofloxacin, and these compounds have enjoyed considerable clinical success. However, some species, such as *Staphylococcus aureus*, *Pseudomonas aeruginosa*, and *Mycobacterium tuberculosis*, acquire resistance mutations that limit fluoroquinolone usefulness. Topoisomerase-based resistance to the fluoroquinolones occurs in a stepwise manner, with moderate levels arising from single mutations in the primary target of the drug (gyrase or topoisomerase IV, depending on the bacterial species). Higher levels of resistance result from additional mutations in both the primary and secondary targets. In Gram-positive organisms such as *S. aureus*, first-step mutations occur in *parC* while second step alleles map in *gyrA*. The situation is reversed in Gram-negative bacteria. For example, with *Neisseria gonorrhoeae* the first two stepwise mutations occur in *gyrA*, and the next two occur in *parC*. This quinolone target difference between the two organisms arises largely because gyrase of Gram-positive bacteria is much less susceptible to attack by the quinolones than gyrase of Gram-negative species.

Computer-based studies indicate that alkoxy or halogen substituents at the C-8 position of N-1 cyclopropyl fluoroquinolones are likely to increase inhibitory activity against *S. aureus, P. aeruginosa,* and mycobacteria. Since quinolones containing C-8 halogens tend to exhibit unacceptable side effects, most of the attention has focused on C-8-methoxy derivatives. Early studies with *E. coli* were not very promising when bacteriostatic action was examined: a C-8-methoxy compound was less effective than a C-8-hydrogen derivative against wild-type cells. This was also true for a first-step resistant *gyrA* mutant, but the difference between the compounds was much less. Since lethal action is a separate event from blocking growth, we also compared the compounds for their ability to kill cells. By this assay the C-8-methoxy compound was more effective against both wild-type and mutant cells [3]. This result was encouraging because we anticipated that highly lethal compounds would make bacterial populations less likely to acquire resistance arising from the mild mutagenic action of the SOS response.

We next tested C-8-methoxy compounds against wild-type and *gyrA* mutants of mycobacteria. With *Mycobacterium bovis* BCG, a C-8 methoxy group doubled bacteriostatic action against wild-type cells and increased it by a factor of ten when a first-step *gyrA* mutant was examined [5]. The C-8-methoxy group also increased lethal action against wild-type and mutant cells (Fig. 2).

Results with *M. bovis* BCG were extended to multidrug-resistant isolates of *M. tuberculosis* that had been obtained from patients who had been unsuccessfully treated with ciprofloxacin. These *gyrA* mutants exhibited increased resistance to ciprofloxacin [6]. When examined in broth culture, the resistant mutants were more readily killed by a C-8-methoxy compound than by its C-8-hydrogen control or ciprofloxacin [7]. The C-8-methoxy compounds were also more lethal when these *M. tuberculosis* isolates infected cultured macrophages [7]. Thus the

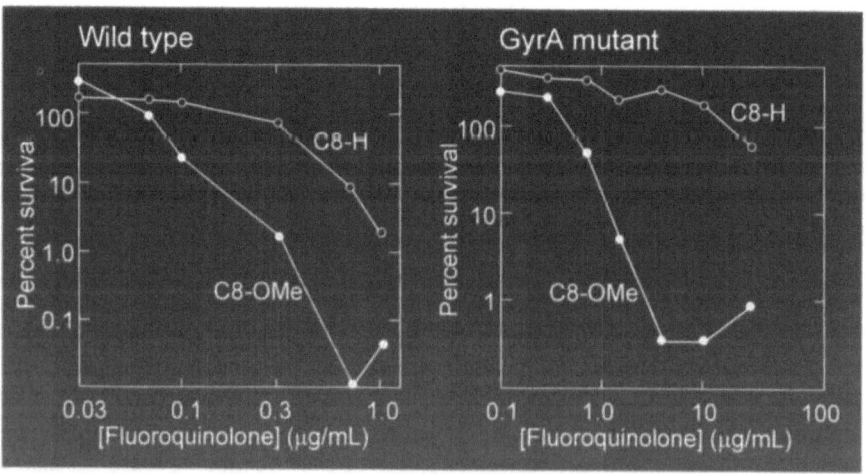

Fig. 2. Effect of a C-8 methoxy group on the bactericidal action of fluoroquinolones against *Mycobacterium bovis* BCG

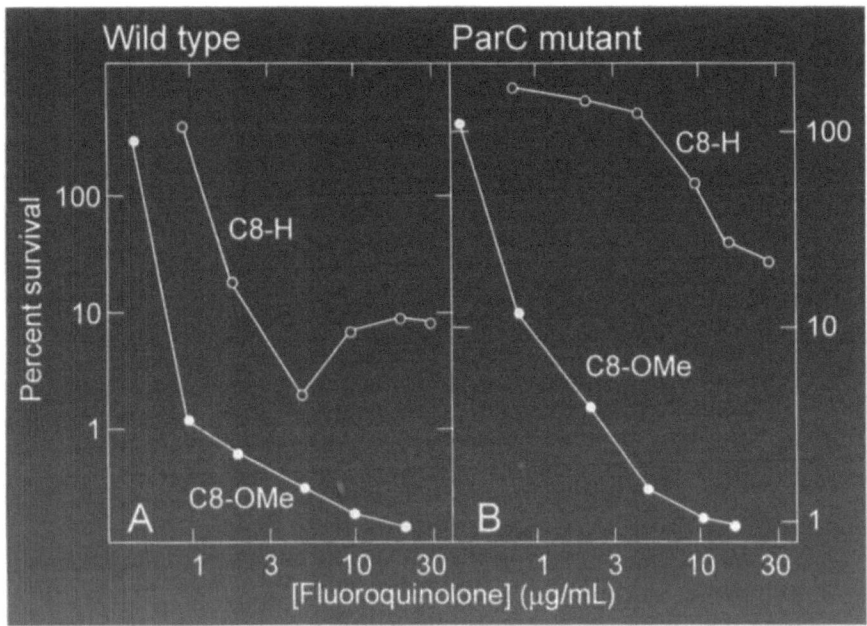

Fig. 3. Effect of a C-8 methoxy group on the bactericidal action of fluoroquinolones against *Staphylococcus aureus*

C-8-methoxy group may help make fluoroquinolones more effective anti-tuberculosis agents.

The C-8-methoxy substituent also improved the bactericidal activity of fluoroquinolones against wild-type *S. aureus* (Fig. 3) [8]. Relative to its C-8-hydrogen control, the C-8-methoxy compound was even more effective against a first-step *parC* mutant. Thus the C-8-methoxy group improves lethal activity against both gyrase and topoisomerase IV.

Since the C-8-methoxy compounds were particularly active against resistant mutants, we expected the compounds to restrict the ability of bacterial populations to become resistant because outgrowth of resistant mutants would be prevented. As an initial test of this idea, we plated dense cultures, on the order of 10^{10} cells, on agar plates containing C-8-methoxy or C-8-hydrogen fluoroquinolones. Concentrations were found at which a thousand colonies were recovered from plates containing the C-8-hydrogen compounds while none were found on plates containing the C-8-methoxy derivatives [5]. As shown in Table 1, this was true for several bacterial species.

We expected that a concentration window would exist in which mutants could be obtained from cell cultures when challenged by a C-8-hydrogen compound but not by a C-8-methoxy derivative. To examine this idea we plated cells on agar containing various concentrations of fluoroquinolone [9]. As we increased the concentration, the number of colonies recovered from agar plates dropped sharply when the MIC was exceeded, presumably due to the inhibition of wild-

Table 1
Restricted selection of
resistant mutants by
C-8-methoxy fluoroquino-
lones. About 10^{10} cells of the
indicated bacterial species
were applied to agar plates
containing C-8-methoxy or
C-8-hydrogen fluoroquino-
lones. After appropriate
incubation the number of
colonies arising on the plates
were counted

Compound	Resistant mutants recovered
Escherichia coli	
Ciprofloxacin (C8-H)	1,700
PD135042 (C8-OMe)	0
Mycobacterium smegmatis	
PD160793 (C8-H)	1,100
PD161148 (C8-OMe)	0
Mycobacterium bovis BCG	
PD160793 (C8-H)	1,052
PD161148 (C8-OMe)	0
Mycobacterium tuberculosis	
PD160793 (C8-H)	1,334
PD161148 (C8-OMe)	0

type growth. At about three times the MIC, the response leveled off, and a distinct plateau was observed. The plateau was probably due to the presence of resistant mutants in the population. At very high concentration, the recovery of mutants again dropped sharply. At this point the MIC of the most resistant first-step mutant had been exceeded. At concentrations above the MIC of first-step mutants it was difficult to recover resistant mutants, since a rare double mutation would be required to attain a level of resistance sufficient to overcome the quinolone. The point at which no mutants are recovered we call the mutant prevention concentration (MPC). The C-8-methoxy group lowers the fluoroquinolone concentration required to achieve the MPC (Fig. 4).

Measurement of MPC provides a new way to evaluate quinolone potency. In practice, MPC can be determined by employing the same agar dilution method used for MIC determination. The difference is that many more cells, on the order of 10^{10}, are applied to agar plates to measure MPC. Thus it is generally necessary to concentrate the cells by centrifugation prior to plating. Since MPC is determined using wild-type bacterial populations, it is not necessary to have first-step resistant mutants available. Consequently, the method is easily applied to any bacterium that can be plated in large numbers. For comparative purposes, it is necessary to qualify the number, since MPC is influenced by the number of cells tested. We generally indicate the number of cells tested as a subscript as in MPC_{1010}.

In addition to being useful for identifying compounds that are least likely to select resistant mutants, MPC also helps define therapeutic doses that will restrict the development of resistance in patients. Such a parameter may be particularly useful for cases in which patients are immunocompromised.

In the work described above, the focus was on very high concentrations of quinolone. Another approach, which has been taken by Professor A. Dalhoff of Bayer AG, is to examine the ability of compounds to delay the development of resistance when cells are challenged with low doses [10]. In an experiment with *S. aureus*, Dalhoff first performed standard MIC determinations with 2-fold dilutions. He then took cells from the highest concentration that allowed growth

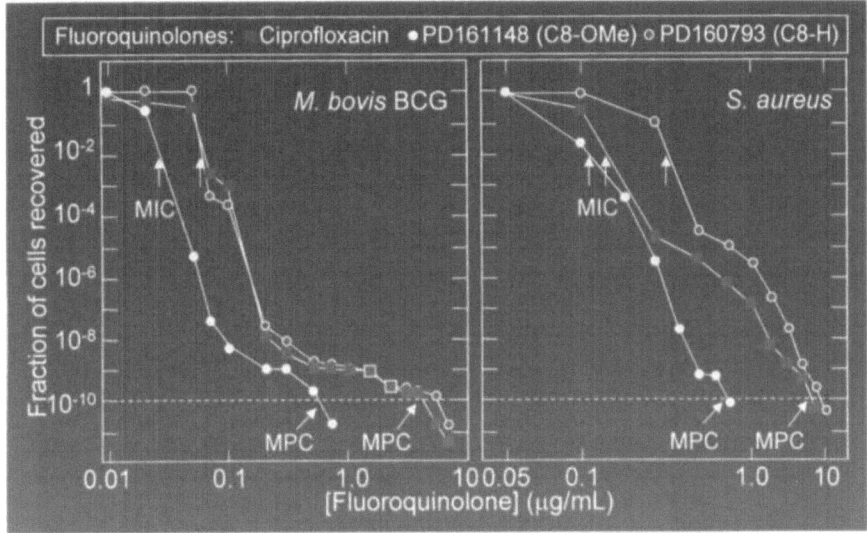

Fig. 4. Effect of fluoroquinolone concentration on the selection of resistant mutants of *Mycobacterium bovis* BCG and *Staphylococcus aureus*

Fig. 5
Effect of multiple challenges
on the development of
fluoroquinolone resistance in
Staphylococcus aureus

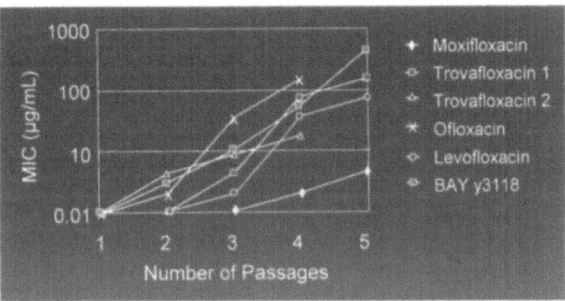

(0.5 times MIC) and performed another MIC determination. This process was repeated several times to determine the number of passages that would occur before the population displayed high-level resistance. When several fluoroquinolones were examined, *S. aureus* required more rounds of challenge to acquire resistance with moxifloxacin, a C-8-methoxy compound, than with ofloxacin, levofloxacin, or trovafloxacin (Fig. 5). Thus C-8-methoxy fluoroquinolones restrict gradual, step-wise selection of resistance as well as the one-step acquisition of high-level resistance.

Conclusions

The C-8-methoxy fluoroquinolones, of which moxifloxacin is an example, have the unusual ability to avidly attack resistant mutants. This is true at both the bacteriostatic and bactericidal level for *E. coli, S. aureus,* and *M. tuberculosis.* Consequently, the C-8-methoxy compounds restrict the selection of resistant mutants by bacterial populations. We currently view fluoroquinolones with C-8 substituents as a special subgroup of the quinolones, and we expect these compounds to be exceptional antibacterial agents.

References

1. Drlica K, Zhao X (1997) DNA gyrase, topoisomerase IV, and the 4-quinolones. Microbiol and Molec Biol Reviews 61:377–392
2. Khodursky A, Cozzarelli N (1998) The mechanism of inhibition of topoisomerase IV by quinolone antibacterials. J Biol Chem 273:27668–27677
3. Zhao X, Xu C, Domagala J, Drlica K (1997) DNA topoisomerase targets of the fluoroquinolones: a strategy for avoiding bacterial resistance. Proc Natl Acad Sci USA 94:13991–13996
4. Chen C-R, Malik M, Snyder M, Drlica K (1996) DNA gyrase and topoisomerase IV on the bacterial chromosome: quinolone-induced DNA cleavage. J Mol Biol 258:627–637
5. Dong Y, Xu C, Zhao X, Domagala J, Drlica K (1998) Fluoroquinolone action against mycobacteria: effects of C8 substituents on bacterial growth, survival, and resistance. Antimicrob Agents Chemother 42:2978–2984
6. Xu C, Kreiswirth BN, Sreevatsan S, Musser JM, Drlica K (1996) Fluoroquinolone resistance associated with specific gyrase mutations in clinical isolates of multidrug resistant *Mycobacterium tuberculosis.* J Infect Disease 174:1127–1130
7. Zhao B-Y, Pine R, Domagala J, Drlica K (1999) Fluoroquinolone action against clinical isolates of *Mycobacterium tuberculosis*: effects of a C8-methoxyl group on survival in liquid media and in human macrophages. Antimicrob Agents Chemother 43:661–666
8. Zhao X, Wang J-Y, Xu C, Dong Y, Zhou J, Domagala J, Drlica K (1998) Killing of *Staphylococcus aureus* by C-8-methoxy fluoroquinolones. Antimicrob Agents Chemother 42:956–958
9. Dong Y, Zhao X, Domagala J, Drlica K (1999) Effect of fluoroquinolone concentration on selection of resistant mutants of *Mycobacterium bovis* BCG and *Staphylococcus aureus.* Antimicrob Agents Chemother 43:1756–1758
10. Dalhoff A (1998) Dissociated resistance among fluoroquinolones. EEC Hamburg.

Discussion on Mechanisms of Fluoroquinolone Resistance

QUESTION: Dr. Drlica, how do you control your experiments, given the fact that some of these quinolones may themselves promote mutations? It has been postulated that ciprofloxacin, for instance, may produce adapted mutation, increasing the rate of mutation towards the compound. I wonder if some of these differences you have found are not differences based on the ability or lack of ability of some compounds to provoke adaptive mutation.

ANSWER: This is currently under study. Quinolone-induced mutations are most easily studies in *E. coli* where, for instance, you have *LexA* mutants in which you can block the SOS response. It is very difficult to get at this question directly. I think the important point that comes out of your question, though, is that it is important to kill cells, rather than simply block their growth. What I would like to stress is that the compounds that are very good at killing are probably those that we should look at especially closely.

QUESTION: Would your concept of MPC confirm that we have been under-dosing for a long period of time and that we should give higher doses in order to prevent the appearance of mutations?

ANSWER: Yes, I think that what you need to do is be above the MIC of the most resistant first-step mutant, which is the MPC. Usually for any random organism that we have heard about here today, you do not have first-step mutants to study. You do not know what genes they map in. But you can generate the kind of curve that we show. For it you do not have to know anything about the first-step mutants. If you measure MPC with a lot of cells, it does not matter whether it is a pump mutation or a gyrase or a topoisomerase IV mutation. If you are above the MPC, you are not getting any mutants. That will prevent new resistant populations from arising.

CHAPTER 15

Pre-clinical Microbiology – Summary II   **15**

BERND WIEDEMANN

The preceding reviews of pre-clinical microbiology can be summarised as follows:

Dr. Gillespie dealt with *Mycobacteria*. He indicated that moxifloxacin is active in vitro against *M. tuberculosis* and *M. avium*. In-vitro studies show that moxifloxacin achieves adequate intracellular killing and animal models support these findings.

Dr. Goldstein showed that moxifloxacin is also active against a wide variety of anaerobic species, from *Bacteroides* to peptostreptococci. Moxifloxacin may be useful in a variety of infections where anaerobes are implicated, from abdominal to dental infections and those resulting from bites. Moxifloxacin's minimal activity versus *C. difficile* may be a benefit, although this needs further confirmation.

Fastidious Gram-negative organisms were covered by Dr. Bauernfeind, who explained that moxifloxacin, like other quinolones, is highly active against *Haemophilus*, *Neisseria*, *Moraxella* and *Pasteurella*.

The susceptibility of respiratory tract isolates to antimicrobials was reviewed by Dr. Sahm. Resistance among American *Haemophilus* and *Moraxella* are maintained at high levels, 33% and 92% of the isolates, respectively, produced beta-lactamase. Pneumococcal resistance continues to increase, not only to beta-lactams but also to macrolides, tetracyclines and trimethoprim-sulpha, but not to fluoroquinolones. Regional variability in resistance is observed, so one needs to be aware of the local situation e.g. resistance of *S. pneumoniae* to penicillin is 24% in southeastern USA and 12% in northeastern USA.

Dr. Felmingham continued the review of RTI susceptibility from an EU perspective. He commented on the remarkable variations seen within a country (e.g. France), and between adjacent countries (e.g. France and Germany). Antibiotic consumption clearly drives resistance, though this may be related to more than just amount, but also to the per patient dosing and duration.

Dr. Tomono concluded the section on RTI susceptibility surveys with some additional points. Japan is a very heavy "consumer" of antibiotics, but resistance is not particularly worse than elsewhere. There are, however, still the same issues of resistance. In Japan, *S. pneumoniae* are about 25% resistant to penicillin. *H. influenzae* is around 15% resistant to ampicillin, and based on data from Nagasaki, *M. catarrhalis* strains are 100% resistant to ampicillin.

Finally, the mechanisms of fluoroquinolone action and resistance were elucidated by Dr. Drlica. It appears that there are two sites of fluoroquinolone activity, and there is exquisite sensitivity of an organism to specific fluoro-quinolones, thus not all fluoroquinolones are the same. Structure-activity relationship studies have been used to improve fluoroquinolone activity at the specific molecular level (e.g. C-8 methoxy). With regard to dissociated quinolone resistance, individual fluoroquinolones do vary in their ability to select for resistance. Add this phenomenon to the pharmacodynamic attributes of a quinolone, and it should be possible to prescribe an agent that not only confers clinical efficacy, but also reduces the selection pressure which drives antibiotic resistance development.

Part 3
Pharmacology

CHAPTER 16

Pharmacokinetics and Pharmacodynamics of Antimicrobials

16

RICHARD WISE

Abstract. The pharmacology of beta-lactams, macrolides, aminoglycosides and fluoroquinolones will be discussed in terms of their bioavailability, protein binding, volume of distribution, tissue penetration and elimination. The high volume of distribution of the quinolones differentiates this class of agents from the others and highlights their high tissue distribution. The penetration into important sites of the body is fundamental to their clinical efficacy. For example, the fluoroquinolones penetrate the tissues of the respiratory tract and concentrate in the bronchial mucosa, the epithelial lining and the alveolar macrophages. The pharmacokinetics and the high in-vitro activity of this group of compounds underpins their broad clinical use.

This chapter will deal with the pharmacology of the four major classes of antimicrobials, beta-lactams, macrolides, aminoglycosides and fluoroquinolones, with special reference to moxifloxacin.

Pharmacodynamics

Most discussion of pharmacodynamics will be left for subsequent chapters, but one aspect that will be mentioned is post-antibiotic effect. This is the phenomenon where an antimicrobial appears to be exerting its effect well after its concentration has fallen below the MIC level. The post-antibiotic effect may be related to a lag-time in the regeneration of the target site after it has been 'hit' by the antimicrobial. The beta-lactams have a reasonable post-antibiotic effect, up to about three hours in Gram-positive bacteria, less so in Gram-negative organisms. The macrolides, also have a post-antibiotic effect ranging between 1.5 to 4 h in Gram-positive cocci. The aminoglycosides have a shorter post-antibiotic effect as do the fluoroquinolones (2 and 2–3 h, respectively). This post-antibiotic effect is most important for the beta-lactams due to their short elimination half-lives of about 1 h. If their effect is prolonged by up to a further 3 h, this represents a significant increase. For the fluoroquinolones which have much longer half-lives, the post-antibiotic effect is a less relevant pharmacodynamic parameter.

Pharmacokinetics

Absorption

Beta-lactams are known to have highly variable absorption. Some beta-lactams, such as cephalexin and cephradine, are almost 100% orally absorbed. Others are so poorly absorbed (e.g. cefuroxime) that pro-drugs must be used to aid their absorption. The macrolide drugs are also variably absorbed. For instance, bioavailability for clarithromycin and roxithromycin is good, while that for erythromycin and dirythromycin is poor. The aminoglycosides, of course, have negligible absorption, while fluoroquinolone absolute bioavailability is high and ranges from approximately 50% for rufloxacin to greater than 85% for most of the other fluoroquinolones.

Protein binding

In terms of protein binding, most fluoroquinolones are not highly bound. Moxifloxacin is only 30–40% bound, gatifloxacin and levofloxacin, slightly less so, clinafloxacin slightly more, with trovafloxacin showing the highest protein binding (70–80%). This is relevant because the higher the binding, the less antimicrobial activity in the presence of serum. Thus, if one antimicrobial is 0% bound and another is 50% bound, the second drug will be half as active in the presence of serum. Protein binding also affects tissue penetration. Penetration is lower with a higher bound agent.

The effect of protein binding on beta-lactam tissue penetration was investigated using the blister fluid model [1]. Figure 1 plots peak blister fluid levels of free antibiotic against the protein binding of the drug in that fluid. The results illustrate the relationship between protein binding and beta-lactam penetration; the higher the protein binding, the lower the tissue penetration.

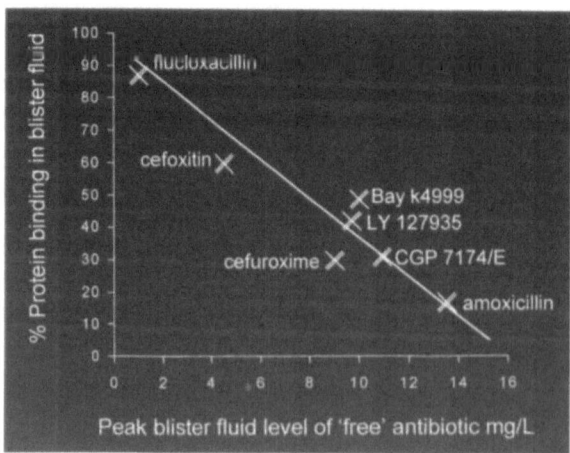

Fig. 1
The relationship between protein binding and beta lactam penetration using the blister fluid model

Distribution

Antimicrobial tissue penetration is usually judged by volume of distribution. Beta-lactams and aminoglycosides have a low volume of distribution (0.18 – 0.25 L/kg). Their distribution is mostly limited to the circulating blood volume and perhaps the highly perfused organs of the body. Macrolides and fluoroquinolones have higher volumes of distribution (1 – 2 and 3 L/kg, respectively) and this represents an important therapeutic property.

Beta-lactams are essentially confined to extravascular space, therefore, one must use very high doses to 'push' them into tissue compartments. Fortunately, these are relatively safe drugs, and this approach can be used successfully. Aminoglycosides have similar properties though they are somewhat dose-limited by their toxicity. Macrolides have good tissue penetration, especially azithromycin, and the fluoroquinolones have particularly good penetration.

It is the high volume of distribution that provides fluoroquinolones with their pharmacokinetic opportunities and these in turn produce clinical opportunities. Figure 2 illustrates some of the known sites of tissue distribution for fluoroquinolones. They are rapidly and completely absorbed into the bloodstream and from there they quickly penetrate into extracellular fluid, phagocytes and into mucosa. The mucosa is essentially the difference between the inside of the body and the outside of the body and this is the site of many infections. Fluoroquinolones are concentrated two to three-fold vs. plasma at these mucosal sites.

Studies comparing fluoroquinolone penetration using the inflammatory (blister) fluid model [2, 3, 4] showed that moxifloxacin, ciprofloxacin, gatifloxacin, sparfloxacin and norfloxacin penetration ranged from 107 to 117%. Trovafloxacin had the lowest penetration (63%) which was probably related to its higher protein binding.

For effective antimicrobial therapy, it is important that concentrations reach significant intracellular concentrations. Most beta-lactams do not reach these levels, nor do aminoglycosides. Macrolides, fluoroquinolones and tetracyclines, on the other hand, all show good intracellular penetration and reach significant intracellular concentrations.

Fig. 2
The sites of fluoroquinolone distribution

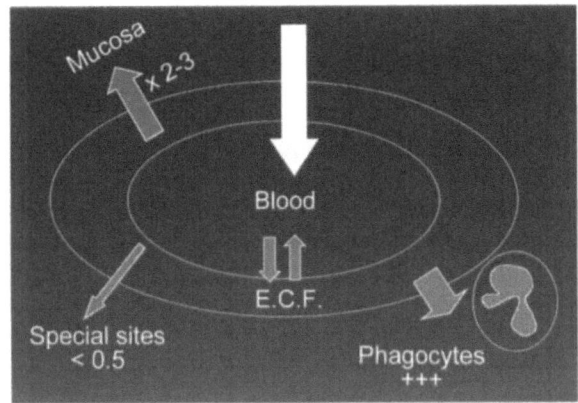

Table 1
The penetration of selected
antibiotics into cerebrospinal
fluid in the rabbit meningitis
model

	%	
Penicillins	5–10	
Cephalosporins	5–10	
Meropenem	21	} T/2 > serum
Gentamicin	0–30	
Vancomycin	7–14	
Ciprofloxacin	26	
Trovafloxacin	23	} T/2 = serum
Ofloxacin	42–72	

Another site that is clinically relevant is the cerebrospinal fluid (CSF). One study compared the penetration of several antimicrobials into CSF in the rabbit meningitis model and the results are shown in Table 1 [3]. One interesting discovery was that drugs such as the cephalosporins, penetrated poorly into the CSF but once there, they tended to linger. Their half-life within the CSF was considerably greater than in serum. The fluoroquinolones, however, seemed to get in and out rapidly and their half-life in the CSF was similar to that of serum.

To summarize, fluoroquinolones are widely distributed throughout the body with the exception of the CNS and perhaps the anterior chamber of the eye. Most fluoroquinolones have low protein binding, which accounts for the high intracellular penetration and large volume of distribution.

Elimination

The majority of beta-lactams are renally excreted, with a few notable exceptions such as ceftriaxone and cefoperazone, which also have significant biliary excretion. Most macrolides exhibit extensive metabolism. Erythromycin, clarithromycin and azithromycin are all N-demethylated, other macrolides such as clarithromycin are extensively hydroxylated. The aminoglycosides, on the other hand, are completely eliminated by the renal route. Fluoroquinolones can be eliminated by renal or faecal routes, or trans-intestinally across the GI tract. Fluoroquinolone metabolism also occurs and is associated with the C7 position. If this metabolism is cytochrome P_{450}-related, then drug interactions may be of concern.

The rate of elimination is an important pharmacokinetic parameter for any drug. Beta-lactams generally have short half-lives; 20 min for benzyl penicillin, 50 min for cefaclor. Hence, the requirement for 2–4, or more, doses per day. For the macrolides, azithromycin has a longer half-life than clarithromycin and erythromycin has the shortest half-life (1.5 h). Aminoglycoside half-lives range from 2–3 h, therefore, based on pharmacokinetics, one would think that they should be administered several times a day. In fact the drugs are only given once daily because they seem to kill bacteria in a concentration-independent fashion.

Fluoroquinolone half-lives vary from 4–5 h for ciprofloxacin, through 6–7 h for levofloxacin, to 10–14 h for moxifloxacin and trovafloxacin. Therefore ciprofloxacin and levofloxacin should be administered twice a day. The newer agents such as moxifloxacin, trovafloxacin, gemifloxacin, have longer half lives and are true once-daily drugs.

The elimination profiles for fluoroquinolones vary greatly. Two thirds of ciprofloxacin elimination is non-renal (metabolism and trans-intestinal), while some drugs such as levofloxacin are almost entirely renally excreted (80% to 90%). These differences are significant because highly metabolised drugs have a potential for 'metabolic' drug interactions. Those that have high metabolic or renal excretion may also need dose adjustment in patients with excretory organ failure. Most of the other fluoroquinolones are not cause for concern, because they have more than one route of excretion.

Conclusion

The fluoroquinolones have the most desirable pharmacokinetic properties of all the major groups of antimicrobials. They have rapid and complete absorption, high tissue penetration and elimination rates that suggest once daily dosing. Differences are now appearing amongst the fluoroquinolones in such aspects as metabolism and protein binding. These features should be used to determine preferences between drugs.

References

1. Wise R, Gillet P, Cadge B, Durnham SR, Baker S (1980) The influence of protein binding upon the tissue fluid levels of 6 Beta-lactam antibiotics. J Infect Dis 142:77–82
2. Wise R. in Press
3. Johnson JH, Cooper MA, Andrews JM, Wise R (1992) Pharmacokinetics and inflammatory fluid penetration of sparfloxacin. Antimicrobial Agents and Chemotherapy 36(11):2444–2446
4. Wise R, Mortiboy D, Child J, Andrews JM (1996) Pharmacokinetics and penetration into inflammatory fluid of trovafloxacin (CP-99,219). Antimicrobial Agents and Chemotherapy 40(1):47–49
5. Lutsar et al. (1998) In: Programme and Abstracts of the Eight International Conference on Infectious Diseases, Boston, MA 1998

CHAPTER 17

Mini-Reviews – Pharmacokinetics/Pharmacodynamics (PK/PD)

17

JEROME J. SCHENTAG

Abstract. The pharmacokinetic and pharmacodynamic aspects of antimicrobials can be integrated using the AUIC, which is the AUC_{24}/MIC. Based on a study in patients with nosocomial pneumonia, a ciprofloxacin AUIC < 125 did not eradicate the pathogen in 2/3 of patients. An AUIC > 250 produced the most rapid and complete eradication. Experience has shown that the pathogens with MIC values below the AUIC value of 100 are responsible for the emergence of resistance. Therefore, resistance can be avoided by adequately exceeding the AUIC of 100 with those pathogens. Most rapid killing of organisms can be achieved with AUIC target values of 250.

Introduction

Up until now we have reviewed the microbiology of antimicrobial drugs, particularly moxifloxacin, and we have also been introduced to their pharmacokinetics. My role will be to put these two aspects together. I will begin with a few introductory remarks, to focus the presenters that will continue the PK/PD discussion in more detail.

Results and Discussion

Figure 1 describes the pharmacokinetics of 400 mg of moxifloxacin following once daily dosing [1]. At steady-state, the peak serum concentration for one dosing interval is 2.5 µg/mL and the area under the curve (AUC_{24}) is approximately 35 µg · h/mL. The figure also shows three possible MIC values represented by three different horizontal lines. The AUIC values represent the ratio of the AUC_{24} to the MIC values.

A MIC value of 1 µg/mL, for instance, would produce an AUIC value of 35. Some investigators think that an AUIC value of 35 denotes borderline efficacy, and this point will be revisited later in the discussion. Clearly, the 0.5 µg/mL MIC value produces better AUIC results, with a peak to MIC ratio of about 5:1 and an AUIC of 70. A MIC value of 0.25 µg/mL produces an AUIC value of 140. A MIC value of 0.125 µg/mL, which is the moxifloxacin MIC_{90} for most respiratory organisms, produces an AUIC value of 280 with a peak to MIC ratio of 20:1. Moxifloxacin appears to be very active because so many of the organisms have low MICs.

It should be kept in mind that the pharmacokinetic data used in this exercise are from normal volunteers, which is usually not an advantage for the drug. In

Fig. 1
The steady-state pharmacokinetics of moxifloxacin following 400 mg q.d. admin-
istration (C_{max}: 2.5 µg/mL,
AUC_{24}: 35 µg · h/mL)

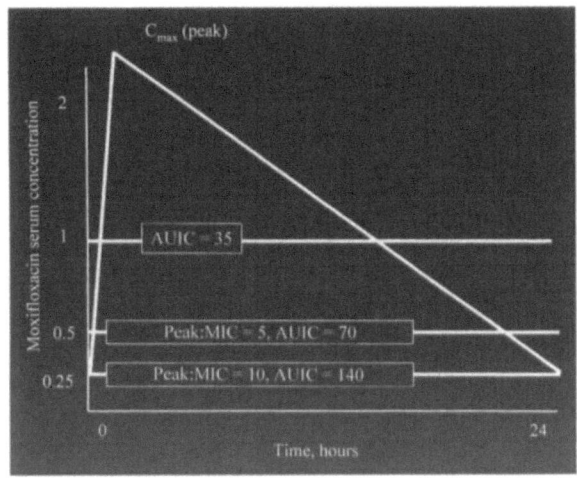

fact, the data from normal volunteers constructs the lowest possible AUC, which
means that the various organ deficiencies and other complications of real
patients, result in higher AUC for real patients, and therefore producing higher
AUIC values than shown in Fig. 1. Second, comparisons are usually based on
MIC_{90} values, which is also the worst possible criterion for evaluating the average potency of the drug. The use of MIC_{90} means that all but 10% of the organisms have a lower MIC value than that used in the calculation. This lowers the
prediction of AUIC. In fact, the important MIC value is not the standardised
value like the MIC_{90}, but the MIC value for that particular patient. Thus, if the
pneumococcus has a MIC_{90} value of 1 µg/mL, but most of the organisms in the
patient are distributed between 0.125 and 0.25 µg/mL, then even a drug with an
AUIC of 35 based on MIC_{90} should produce good results. The only exception
would be for the very few patients who actually are infected with organisms
having the MIC of 1.0 µg/mL.

The lessons taught by ciprofloxacin [2] are particularly useful in understanding the importance of AUIC values (see Fig. 2). Data published in 1993 showed
that a group of patients with nosocomial pneumonia had more rapid eradication of the organism when the ciprofloxacin AUIC value was greater than 250.
The organism was eradicated from more than half of the patients with an AUIC
> 250 on the first day of treatment. When the AUIC was less than 125, the orga-
nisms were eradicated from only about a third of the patients. In the remainder
of patients with AUIC < 125, there were problems because most showed step-
wise increases in MIC values, and most failed to respond clinically. This indicated that they were becoming resistant to treatment. Values between 125 and 250
resulted in the same bacterial endpoint as those with values above 250, but
eradication was much slower. For instance, it took 6 days to get to 50% killing
with an AUIC 125–250, as compared to one day with an AUIC > 250. Thus, from
this study it was learned that an AUIC less than 125 was not desirable and an
AUIC greater than 250 produced best results. Hence, the proposal of an AUIC
breakpoint of 250.

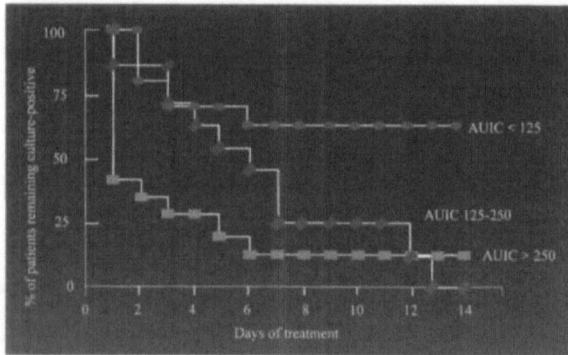

Fig. 2
The relationship between
bacterial eradication
and AUIC in patients with
nosocomial pneumonia

The next stage is to determine the relationship between these dosing concepts and bacterial resistance. It appears that marginal organisms, those with MIC values near the breakpoint, are the ones that cause the problems. They are always the first to start developing the step-wise resistance process, which is now regarded as selective pressure rather than mutation. Resistance is determined by spontaneous mutation rates and the concentration of drug at the site. Emergence by selective pressure occurs when dosing is lowered below the MIC. Therefore, resistance can be avoided by adequately exceeding the MIC of a particular pathogen.

This was demonstrated in a study that followed a large group of patients with nosocomial lower respiratory tract infections [3]. Data are shown in Fig. 3, which plots the probability that the organism would remain susceptible to treatment versus time. Of the patients treated with antimicrobial regimens with AUIC < 100, about half showed step-wise increases in MIC after Day 4. By Day 20, 93 % showed reduced susceptibility. So, virtually all patients with low exposures developed resistance, while only 8 percent of patients with AUIC > 100 did the same.

In terms of antimicrobial exposure, there is also the question of whether one should be dealing with the concentration at the site of action rather than the concentration in the blood. Figure 4 shows a compilation of data from some studies[4,5] which measured the concentrations of moxifloxacin and levofloxacin

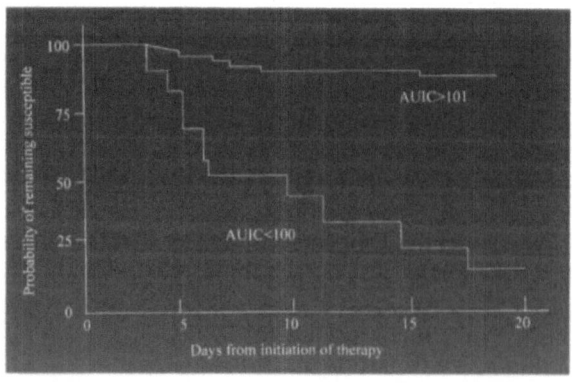

Fig. 3
The relationship between
antimicrobial exposure
(AUIC) and the development
of resistance in patients with
nosocomial lower respiratory
tract infections

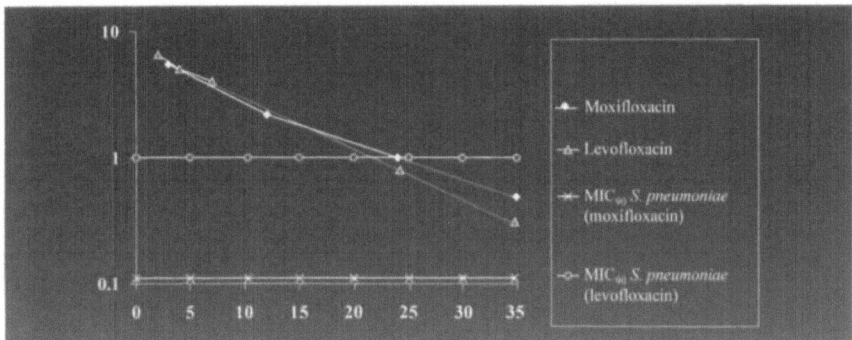

Fig. 4. Concentrations in bronchial mucosa (mg/kg) over time (h) following a single oral dose of moxifloxacin (400 mg) or levofloxacin (500 mg). Dotted lines are extrapolated based on data in references 4 and 5

in bronchial mucosa. Levofloxacin, unlike moxifloxacin, did not provide much coverage above its MIC value in bronchial mucosa. Therefore, concentrations at the site of action should be kept in mind when discussing PK/PD predictions.

Conclusion

Given the points raised in this chapter, I would like our colleagues to ponder a few questions regarding moxifloxacin. First, based on the PK/PD relationship, is bacterial killing predictable for the 400 mg dose chosen for clinical trials? Does this killing occur rapidly in vitro and in vivo? Finally, will the dosage chosen and the use of a very potent agent like moxifloxacin, minimise the risks of resistance in our patients?

References

1. Stass H, Dalhoff A, Kubitza D, Schuhly U (1998) Pharmacokinetics, Safety, and Tolerability of Ascending Doses of Moxifloxacin, a new 8-Methoxy Quinolone, Administered to Healthy Subjects. Antimicrobial Agents and Chemotherapy 42:2060–2065
2. Forest A, Nix DE, Ballow CH, Goss TF, Birmingham MC, Schentag JJ (1993) Pharmacodynamics of intravenous ciprofloxacin in seriously ill patients. Antimicrobial Agents and Chemotherapy 37:1073–1083
3. Thomas JK, Forrest A, Bhavnavi SM, Hyatt JM, Cheng A, Ballow CH, Schentag JJ (1998) Pharmacodynamic evaluation of factors associated with the development of bacterial resistance in acutely ill patients during therapy. Antimicrobial Agents and Chemotherapy 42:521–527
4. Andrews J, Honeybourne D, Jevons G, Wise R (1998) Penetration of moxifloxacin into bronchial mucosa, epithelial lining fluid and alveolar macrophages following a single 400 mg oral dose. In: International Congress of Antimicrobial Agents and Chemotherapy, Abstract A29
5. Andrews JM, Honeybourne D, Jones G, Brunwald NP, Cunningham B, Wise R (1997) Concentration of levofloxacin (HR 355) in the respiratory tract following a single oral dose in patients undergoing fibre-optic in patients undergoing fibre-optic bronchoscopy. Journal of Antimicrobial Chemotherapy 40(4):573–577

In vitro Models as Predictors of the Antimicrobial Effect of Moxifloxacin and Other Fluoroquinolones

STEPHEN ZINNER

Abstract. In-vitro models incorporate pharmacological parameters in the study of antibiotic action. A major advantage over routine in-*vitro* susceptibility testing is the ability to simulate human dosing regimens and apply these changing antibiotic concentrations to the bacterial inoculum. In collaboration with Professor Alexander Firsov of Moscow, we have developed a model that allows the simulation and study of several pharmacokinetic parameters: Area Under the Concentration-Time Curve (AUC), Peak "serum" concentration (C_{max}), time to peak concentration (T_{max}) and elimination half-life ($T_{1/2}$); and pharmacodynamic parameters: AUC/MIC, Time above MIC (T_{eff}), C_{max}/MIC and AUC above the MIC (AUC_{eff}). A new quantitative determinant of antimicrobial effect was defined by Prof. Firsov that describes the area between the control growth curve in the absence of antibiotic and the bacterial killing curve in the presence of antibiotic (Intensity of the effect or I). Moxifloxacin was studied and, at a given AUC/MIC ratio, it produced the largest I_e of five studied fluoroquinolones. Relating various pharmacodynamic predictors to the antimicrobial effect (I_e) suggests that AUC/MIC is the best comparative predictor of the fluoroquinolone antimicrobial effect. Direct comparative studies with levofloxacin suggest that at any AUC/MIC ratio ≥ 100, moxifloxacin produced a greater I_e; a 400 mg daily dose of moxifloxacin was more efficient than 500 mg levofloxacin against a susceptible strain of *Staphylococcus aureus*.

This chapter will examine the value of in-vitro models as predictors of antimicrobial effect.

Most in-vitro models tend to be continuous culture systems with a variety of filters and capillary units, or chambers into which antibiotics are pumped to mimic the concentration of these drugs in human subjects. These studies can be used to add pharmacologic parameters to in-vitro determinations of antimicrobial effects. They may also be useful in antimicrobial pre-clinical development, suggesting doses or schedules to be studied in the clinic. One or more drugs with similar or differing pharmacokinetics can be compared using appropriate in-vitro models.

Figure 1 is the schematic of an in vitro model, with artificial capillary units reflecting the peripheral compartment of a two-compartment model. Drugs are pumped into the central compartment, diluted to simulate the half-life of the drug and then pumped rapidly to the organisms in the small chambers. One-compartment models have also been used successfully.

Some of the many pharmacokinetic and pharmacodynamic parameters that can be studied using these models have already been explained. The parameters include the area under the concentration-time curve (AUC), the peak concentration (C_{max}), the time concentrations that are above the MIC (T_{eff}), the half-life ($t_{1/2}$), and finally the AUIC, which is AUC/MIC [1].

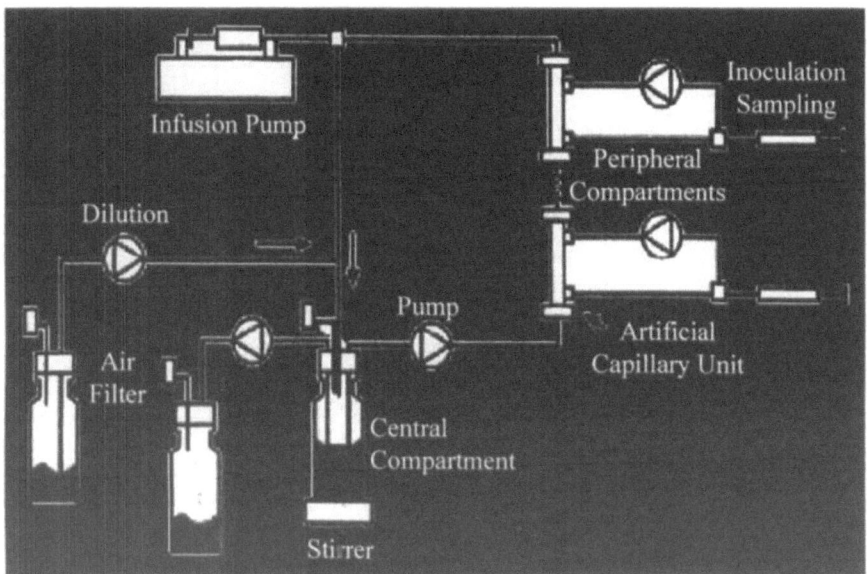

Fig. 1. A two-compartment kinetic model for multiple cultures

On the bacterial side, there are many end points of antimicrobial effect (AME). One can measure the time to reduce the initial inoculum by either 99 or 99.9 percent (T_{99} or $T_{99.9}$), the actual number of bacteria that are reached at the nadir of the growth curve (log N_{min}), and the difference between the starting inoculum and the minimum inoculum (log N_0 – log N_{min}). Other parameters include the time to achieve the minimum inoculum (T_{min}) and various areas above and below the bacterial curve (AUBC and ABBC). Another proposed parameter describes the intensity of the antimicrobial effect (I_E) [2].

Figure 2 illustrates some of the different antimicrobial effect parameters. The I_E is the area between the control growth curve of bacteria in the absence of antibiotic, and the curve that defines the effect of the drug or bacteria exposed to the antibiotic, following a single simulated in-vitro dose. The larger the difference between the curves, the greater the antimicrobial effect.

The pharmacokinetic profiles of four different fluoroquinolones at four different AUC/MIC ratios were simulated using an in-vitro model. Concentration/MIC versus time curves were plotted for the simulated data (Fig. 3). Results showed four separate curves, representing four different levels of antimicrobial exposure for each fluoroquinolone. Note that differences in slope between drugs primarily reflect differences in half-lives.

Bacterial regrowth occurs after administration of a single dose of antimicrobial. This can be seen in Fig. 4, where the effect of moxifloxacin on *E. coli* and *K. pneumoniae* was plotted for each of the four different AUC/MIC exposures. In the first 10 or 12 hours, it was very difficult to see any difference between drug exposure levels because the bacteria were killed very rapidly. Differences occurred later when bacteria began to regrow. The time to

Fig. 2
Parameters used in the
quantitation of bacterial
killing/regrowth and the
antimicrobial effect

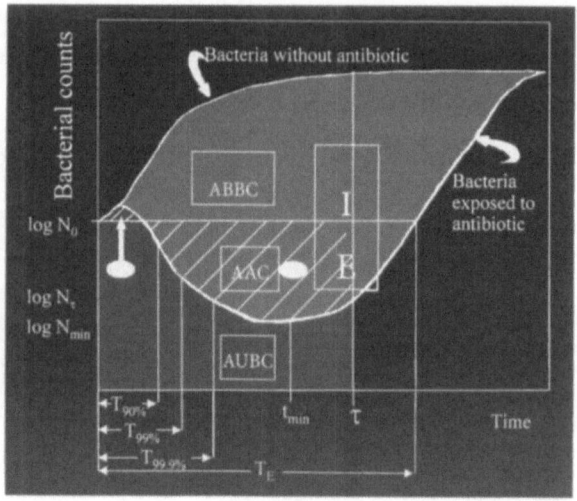

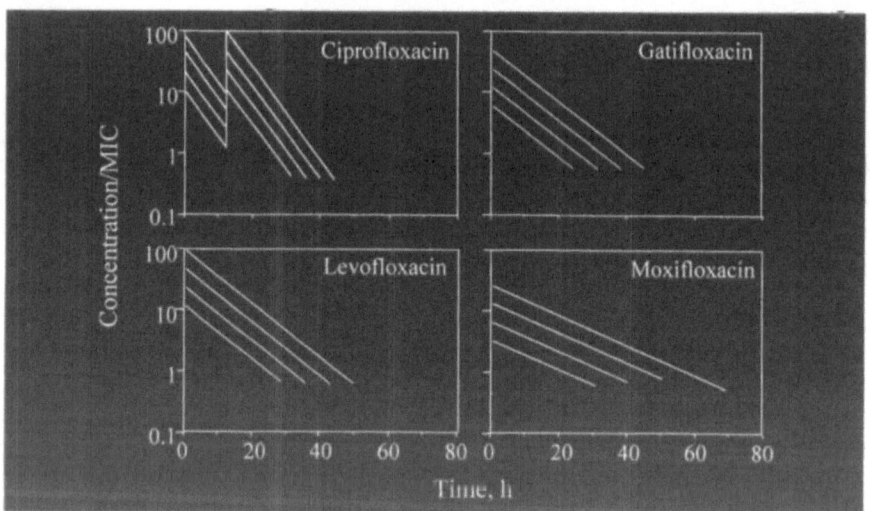

Fig. 3. The in-vitro simulated pharmacokinetic profiles of four fluoroquinolones

regrowth was dependent upon the amount of drug exposure or the AUC/MIC ratio.

Figure 5 is an example of differences in the I_E or the antimicrobial effect parameter. For moxifloxacin, there was a fairly large area, indicating a good effect against S. aureus. The corresponding area for levofloxacin was smaller, so, given similar exposure (AUC/MIC 116 and 117 respectively), the effect against S. aureus was greater for moxifloxacin than for levofloxacin.

When this intensity of effect was plotted vs. the AUC/MIC, curves were produced for each of the fluoroquinolones. The relationship was fluoroquinolone-

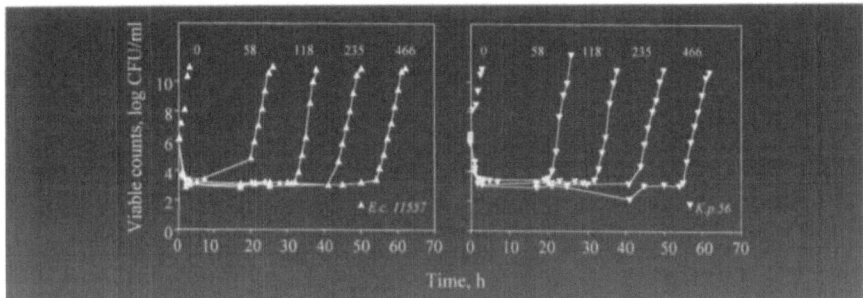

Fig. 4. The kinetics of killing and regrowth of *E. coli* (E. c.) and *K. pneumoniae* (K. p.) exposed to moxifloxacin. The simulated AUC/MIC ratio in [(μg · h/mL)/(μg/mL)] is indicated by the number above each curve

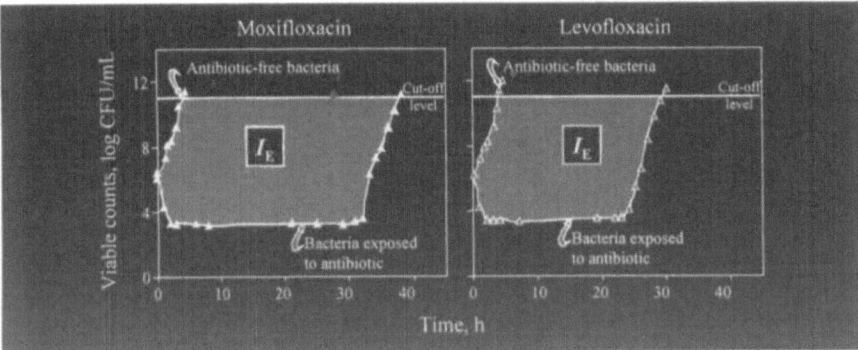

Fig. 5. The kinetics of killing and regrowth of *S. aureus* exposed to moxifloxacin and levofloxacin. AUC/MIC = 117 and 116 (μg · h/mL)/(μg/mL), respectively

specific and appeared to be bacteria-independent. Figure 6 shows the curves for the 4 different compounds. The major difference between these curves is related to half-life. Moxifloxacin has the longest half-life and the steepest AUC/MIC vs. I_E curve, while ciprofloxacin has the shortest half-life and the flattest curve.

At an AUC/MIC ratio of 125 [1], it is clear that the effect obtained with moxifloxacin is greater than that obtained with the other fluoroquinolones. This holds true for virtually all exposure levels and should be of some importance clinically. Another study compared moxifloxacin and levofloxacin activity (I_E) against a number of bacteria at four different exposure (AUC/MIC) levels. Results are summarized in Fig. 7 with exposure plotted versus antimicrobial effect. At an AUC/MIC ratio of 125 moxifloxacin shows approximately 25% greater activity than levofloxacin for all organisms tested.

The next step is to translate the AUC/MIC parameter into dose, and then use the model to predict the dose of moxifloxacin that would produce the same antimicrobial effect as the standard 500 mg dose of levofloxacin. When this was done for *E. coli*, it was determined that 140 mg of moxifloxacin would produce

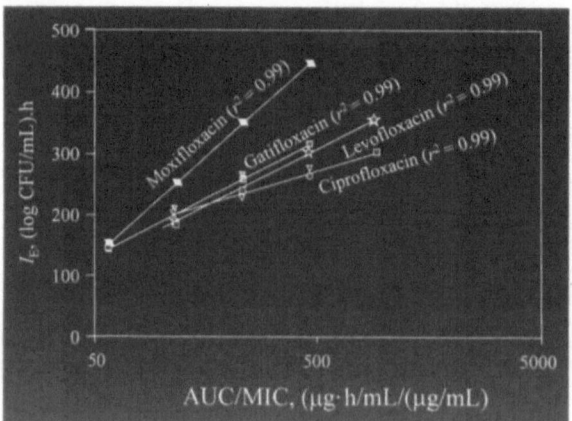

Fig. 6
AUC/MIC-based prediction
of the antimicrobial effects of
fluoroquinolones

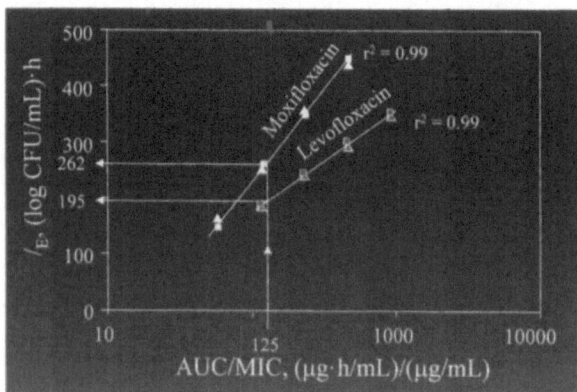

Fig. 7
Dose-dependent antimicro-
bial effects of moxifloxacin
and levofloxacin

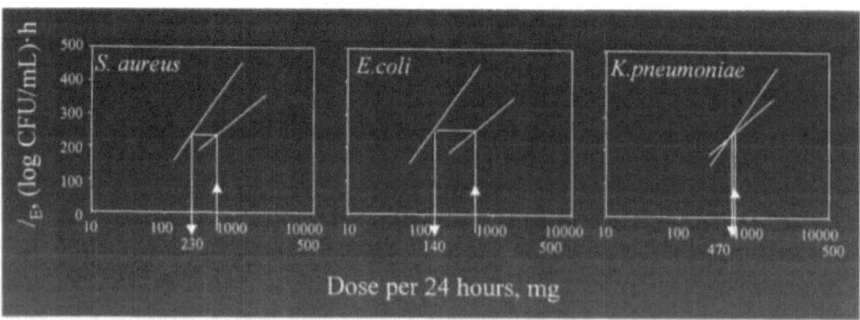

Fig. 8. AUC/MIC-based prediction of the effects of moxifloxacin and levofloxacin on *S. aureus,*
E. coli and *K. pneumoniae*

the same effect as 500 mg of levofloxacin. Similar trends were seen for *S. aureus* and *K. pneumoniae* (see Fig. 8). The model can also be used to predict what dose of levofloxacin would produce the same effect as that obtained with 400 mg moxifloxacin. In-vitro results using a different species of *S. aureus* predicted 1300 mg of levofloxacin would be equi-active to 400 mg of moxifloxacin.

Conclusion

These data suggest that the AUC/MIC parameter is a good intra-quinolone predictor of antimicrobial effect. Of the four fluoroquinolones studied, moxifloxacin produced the largest antimicrobial effect in this model and was clearly more efficient than levofloxacin against *E.coli* and *S. aureus*. So, it can be concluded that in-vitro models are useful in the comparative study of new antibiotics.

References

1. Schentag JJ, Birmingham MC, Paladino JA, Carr JR, Hyatt JM, Forrest A, Zimmer GS, Adelman MH, Cumbo TJ (1997) In nosocomial pneumonia, optimizing antibiotics other than aminoglycosides is a more important determinant of successful clinical outcome, and a better means of avoiding resistance. Semin Respir Infect 12(4):278–293
2. Firsov AA, Vostrov SN, Shevenko AA, Cornaglia G (1997) Parameters of bacterial killing and antimicrobial effect examined in terms of area under the concentration-time curve relationships: action of ciprofloxacin against Escherichia coli in an in-vitro dynamic model. Antimicrobial Agents and Chemotherapy 41:1281–1287

CHAPTER 19

In vitro Models of Infection: Pharmacokinetic/Pharmacodynamic Correlates

ALASDAIR P. MACGOWAN

Abstract. In-vitro models data using simulations of oral 400 mg moxifloxacin, indicate significant bactericidal activity for *S. pneumoniae* strains with MIC ≤ 0.25 µg/mL. Moxifloxacin is also active against *S. aureus* and beta-haemolytic streptococci but has superior activity against *H. influenzae*, *M. catarrhalis* and *K. pneumoniae*. Pharmacodynamic-antibacterial effect correlates are dependent upon the measures of antibacterial effect. Area measures may be superior to log changes in viable count or time to kill a defined percentage of the inoculum. Area-under-the-bacterial-kill-curve (AUBKC) univariate analysis indicates that MIC, T > MIC and AUC/MIC are related to outcome. The relationship between AUC/MIC and transformed AUBKC is described by a sigmoid E_{max} model; the relationship between T > MIC and AUBKC is not. Models to study the combined effects of AUC/MIC and T > MIC indicate the addition of T > MIC to AUC/MIC does not improve the model fit. AUC/MIC is the best parameter in describing the antibacterial effect of moxifloxacin. AUC/MIC ratios based on human pharmacokinetic data and the MIC_{90} of *S. pneumoniae* indicate moxifloxacin should have useful clinical activity.

Introduction

In-vitro pharmacodynamic models of infection are used to perform three types of studies, each with a different function. The first are descriptive studies of antibacterial effect with changing drug concentrations. They determine what effect a simulated dose has on bacterial killing or bacterial clearance from the model. The second type of in-vitro study investigates the effect of changing drug concentrations on the emergence of resistance, and the third attempts to determine pharmacodynamic-antibacterial effect correlates.

Results and Discussion

Table 1 summarises the results of several in-vitro studies which described the antibacterial effect of moxifloxacin [1–5]. Most researchers used the 400 mg dose simulation giving either a single 400 mg dose or two 400 mg doses over a 48-hour period. There was a fair degree of agreement among authors. Results showed significant killing of *S. pneumoniae* when exposed to serum concentrations corresponding to the simulated doses mentioned above (log kill rates ranging 3.5 to 5). Where minimum inhibitory concentration (MIC) values were not reported, wild-type strains with MIC values less than 0.5 or 0.25 µg/mL were

Table 1. A summary of in-vitro studies describing the antibacterial effect of moxifloxacin in *S. pneumoniae*

Simulated dose	Strains		Conclusions	Author
	Numbers	MIC (µg/mgL)		
200 mg × 1	1		<4 log kill	Dalhoff, 1996
400 mg × 2	3	≤0.25	<3.5 log kill	Bowker et al., 1997
	3	≤1.0	>1 log kill	
400 mg × 2	6	0.06–0.5	<5 log kill	Lister et al., 1998
400 mg × 1	6		<4 log kill	Zinner et al., 1998
400 mg × 1	3		<4.5 log kill	Wiedemann, 1998

probably used. Predictably, laboratory-produced resistant strains of *S. pneumoniae* with a moxifloxacin MIC value ≤1 µg/mL showed significantly less killing than wild-type strains (log kill rate <1).

The situation was similar for staphylococci and other kinds of streptococci [1, 6]. All authors described significant drops in viable count after moxifloxacin administration. Dalhoff probably used highly sensitive strains as their log kill rate was <4. Other research performed with Group A Streptococci (GAS) and similar strains of *S. aureus* (Sa) did not show quite the same degree of killing [6].

Figure 1 illustrates how more resistant forms of bacteria produced in the laboratory show less killing. The more sensitive wild-type strains of pneumococcus were rapidly eradicated. Those with slightly higher MIC values had a corresponding slower drop in viable count. While strains with the highest MIC values showed much slower eradication.

Fig. 1
Antibiotic activity against
different strains of
S. pneumoniae

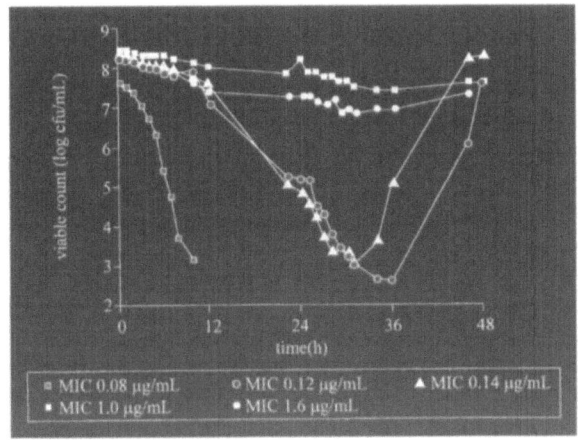

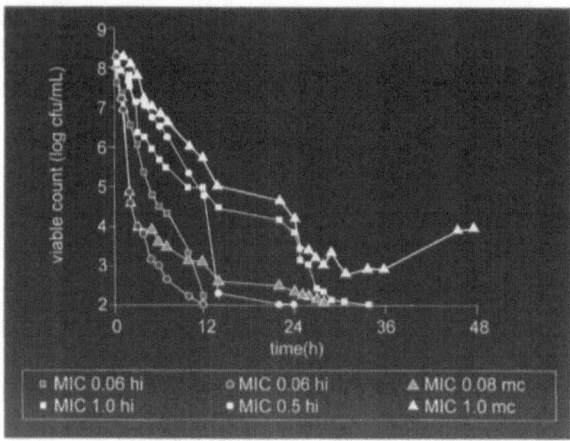

Fig. 2
Antibiotic activity against different strains of *H. influenzae* (hi) and *M. catarrhalis* (mc)

Moxifloxacin, like other fluoroquinolones, shows good activity against Gram-negative bacteria. The in-vitro model was used to test a variety of organisms relevant to respiratory infections such as, *Haemophilus influenzae, Moraxella catarrhalis,* and *Klebsiella pneumoniae.* Again, wild-type strains with low MIC values were rapidly eradicated from these models. Laboratory-produced strains that were a little more resistant showed slower reductions (Fig. 2) [5, 7].

In the next series of experiments, 21 different bacterial strains were used and data were based on a collection of about 70 simulations. This sizeable data set was constructed in order to investigate the pharmacodynamic predictors of bacterial effect. But what measure of antibiotic effect should be used?

The pharmacodynamic factors are more clearly defined: the area under the concentration-time curve divided by the MIC (AUC/MIC), the time that concentrations are above the MIC (T > MIC), and maximum concentration divided by the MIC (C_{max}/MIC).

Figure 2 describes the standard antibacterial effect measures used for in-vitro models. There are many measures, and it is not clear which particular end point should be chosen for a correlation. One could arbitrarily choose the change in viable count at 12 h (Δ12), or perhaps after one dosing interval (Δ24 h). If the in-vitro model runs for 48 h, a 48-hour end point might be appropriate. Many researchers favour looking at the time to produce 2-log and 3-log reductions in count (T99 and T99.9). There are also a number of area measures, such as the area under the bacterial kill curve over 48 h (AUBKC48) or 24 h (AUBKC24). Others prefer to use the area above the bacterial kill curve, which is an equally reasonable choice.

One of the main problems with using measures such as maximum reduction in count (Δ_{max}) is that they are not sensitive for all organisms. Those with low MIC values will not show changes in Δ_{max} after the MIC drops below a threshold value. Once the organism has been totally cleared from the model, it cannot be further cleared. The same holds true for the 'time to kill' parameter. For those organisms with high MIC values, one may never reach a 2-log reduction in

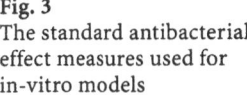

Fig. 3
The standard antibacterial
effect measures used for
in-vitro models

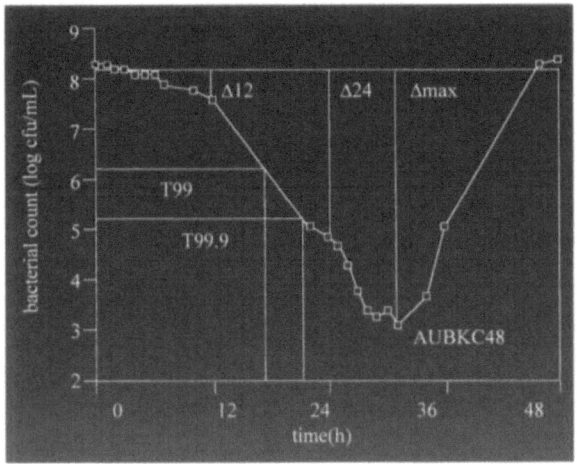

bacterial count. The parameters that do not vary across the whole range of MIC values to be tested are, therefore, not optimal for PK/PD correlation. For example, out of 21 strains tested, the change in viable count at 48 h (Δ48) only varied across the whole range of MIC values on 12 occasions. Consequently this parameter was not very useful.

The only way to properly assess each parameter is to look at variability. Clearly the optimal parameter should be reproducible and this is determined by the % CV (standard deviation/mean × 100). The lower the % CV, the more reproducible the parameter. Based on these criteria, the area parameters showed the best results. They varied best over the full range of MIC values tested and they were the most reproducible parameters for this model.

The parameters of interest, therefore, are based on the area under the bacteria kill curve, which is slightly different to the intensity affect parameter.

Figure 3 shows the relationship between AUBKC and the MIC of the bacteria tested. There appears to be a correlation between these two parameters and the model suggests that moxifloxacin may clear Gram-negative organisms slightly more efficiently than Gram-positive organisms with the same MIC value.

The results of univariate analysis show that the area under the bacterial kill curve (AUBKC24) increases with increasing bacterial MIC. Thus, as expected, there is less killing with more resistant strains. Similarly, as T > MIC increases, or as AUC/MIC increases there is more bacterial killing (AUBKC24 decreases).

The next step is to determine which of these three area parameters is most important. This is clearly difficult to do based on univariate analysis alone. The relationship between AUC and MIC and the antibacterial effect measure can be explored using sigmoidal curve fitting. Experience has shown that it is difficult to get a good fit using T > MIC for fluoroquinolones, however, the AUC/MIC data fit the sigmoid E_{max} model well.

Further statistical tests can be performed looking at the combined effect of the parameters using multivariate analysis. The results showed that the

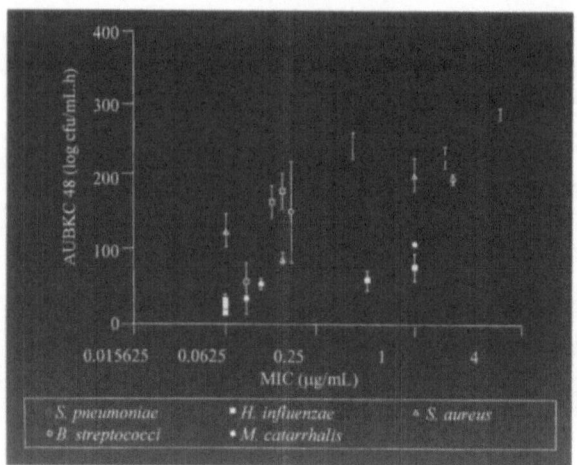

Fig. 4
The relationship between the
MIC and AUBKC parameters

AUC/MIC ratio provided a good fit to AUBKC24, and the addition of T > MIC to the statistical model did not improve fit. Thus, AUC/MIC appears to be the optimal parameter for this particular model.

Table 2 shows the comparative pharmacokinetics of different quinolones and their in-vitro activities against *S. pneumoniae*. It can be seen that, although the kinetics of these drugs do vary somewhat, it is their activity against pneumococci, which shows the most dramatic changes. The comparative pharmacodynamics for the same ten quinolones can be seen in Table 3. Both the AUC/MIC_{90} and C_{max}/MIC_{90} ratios have been proposed as optimal predictors of anti-bacterial effect in man and so these values are presented for comparison. As can be seen, although the two parameters have values of different magnitude, they both produce similar quinolone rankings. Ratios are lowest for lomefloxacin, which is known to have

Table 2. The comparative pharmacokinetics and in-vitro activity of ten fluoroquinolones against *S. pneumoniae* (SpMIC_{90}). Note 3-fold variation in AUC; 4-fold variation in C_{max}; 500-fold variation in MIC_{90}

Agent	Dose (po) (mg)	AUC$_{0-24}$ (µg/mL.h)	C_{max} (µg/mL)	Sp MIC_{90} (µg/mL)
Lomefloxacin	400 OD	32	3.4	16
Ofloxacin	400 BD	42	2.7	2
Ciprofloxacin	750 BD	32	4.0	2
Levofloxacin	500 OD	45	6.0	1
Grepafloxacin	400 OD	15	1.4	0.25
Trovafloxacin	300 OD	39	2.5	0.25
Clinafloxacin	200 BD	45	2.8	0.06
Moxifloxacin	400 OD	34	3.2	0.12
Gatifloxacin	400 OD	30	3.4	0.5
Gemifloxacin	–	–		0.03

Table 3
The comparative pharmaco-
dynamics of ten fluoroquinolones against *S. pneumoniae*

	AUC/MIC$_{90}$	C$_{max}$/MIC$_{90}$
Lomefloxacin	< 5	< 1
Ciprofloxacin Ofloxacin	5 – 25	1 – 5
Levofloxacin Grepafloxacin Gatifloxacin	25 – 75	5 – 10
Trovafloxacin	75 – 250	10 – 20
Moxifloxacin Clinafloxacin Gemifloxacin	> 250	> 20

little activity against *S. pneumoniae*. Drugs such as ciprofloxacin and ofloxacin have ratios ranging from 5–25 for AUC/MIC$_{90}$ and 1–5 for C$_{max}$/MIC$_{90}$. Higher ratios are seen for the more active drugs, levofloxacin, grepafloxacin, gatifloxacin and trovafloxacin. While moxifloxacin, clinafloxacin and gemifloxacin have the highest ratios, > 250 for AUC/MIC$_{90}$ and > 20 for C$_{max}$/MIC$_{90}$.

Conclusion

In conclusion, in-vitro models should use area measures as anti-bacterial end points. The AUC/MIC ratio is the best predictor of anti-bacterial effect as defined by AUBKC. Based on pharmacokinetics and MIC$_{90}$'s against *S. pneumoniae*, moxifloxacin should have significant clinical activity against pneumococci, probably superior to other quinolone comparators.

References

1. Dalhoff A (1996) Antibacterial efficacy of fluctuating concentrations of Bay 12-8039 simulating human serum concentrations. In: Programme and Abstracts of the 36th International Congress of Antimicrobial Agents and Chemotherapy, New Orleans, E26, 104
2. Bowker KE, Wootton M, Holt HA, Reeves DS, MacGowan AP (1998) Bactericidal activity of Bay 12-8039 against *Streptococcus pneumoniae* explored using an in-vitro continuous bactericidal culture model. In: Programme and Abstracts of the 38th International Congress of Antimicrobial Agents and Chemotherapy, San Diego, F134; 169
3. Lister PD, Sanders CC (1998) Pharmacodynamics of moxifloxacin against *Streptococcus pneumoniae* in an in vitro pharmacokinetic model. In: Programme and Abstracts of the 38th International Congress of Antimicrobial Agents and Chemotherapy, San Diego, A21; 7
4. Zinner S, Gilbert D, Simmons K, Sariak E (1998) Moxifloxacin activity against *S. pneumoniae* in an in vitro dynamic model. In: Programme and Abstracts of the 38th International Congress of Antimicrobial Agents and Chemotherapy, San Diego, A26; 8
5. Wiedemann B (1998) Pharmacodynamic activity of moxifloxacin in an in vitro model against Gram-positive and Gram-negative pathogens. In: Programme and Abstracts of the 8th International Conference on Infectious Diseases, Boston, 12.001; 13

6. Wootton M, Bowker KE, Holt HA, MacGowan AP (1998) Bactericidal activity of moxifloxacin against *Staphylococcus aureus* and Group A Streptococci explored using a pharmacodynamic model of infection. In: Programme and Abstracts of the 38th International Congress of Antimicrobial Agents and Chemotherapy, San Diego, A32;10
7. Bowker KE, Wootton M, Holt HA, MacGowan AP (1998) In vitro activity of moxifloxacin against *Haemophilus influenzae* and *Moraxella catarrhalis* investigated using a pharmacodynamic model of infection. In: Programme and A0bstracts of the 38th International Congress of Antimicrobial Agents and Chemotherapy, San Diego, E207; 229

CHAPTER 20

Animal Model Experiences with Moxifloxacin 20

JAMES M. STECKELBERG

Abstract. The efficacy of moxifloxacin in several experimental animal models of infectious diseases was reviewed. In rabbit models of meningitis, treatment with moxifloxacin resulted in a dose-dependent reduction in bacterial density in the CSF; it was equivalent in efficacy to ceftriaxone or vancomycin. In a mouse model of penicillin-resistant streptococcal pneumonia, moxifloxacin was the most effective of the four fluoroquinolones tested. In a murine model of disseminated *Mycobacterium tuberculosis infection,* moxifloxacin, sparfloxacin or isoniazid were equivalent in their ability to prevent mortality and reduce the concentration of bacteria in spleens. Clinafloxacin, although active in vitro, was inactive in vivo in this model. In a rat model of experimental endocarditis caused by methicillin-resistant *Staphylococcus aureus,* moxifloxacin was more effective than ciprofloxacin or vancomycin. The efficacy of moxifloxacin against a ciprofloxacin-resistant strain of MRSA in this model indicated that fluoroquinolone cross-resistance may not be complete. These results indicate moxifloxacin may have a significant clinical role in treating infectious disease.

Introduction

Experimental animal models play an important role in the development and understanding of new antimicrobials. Experimental models have several advantages including the ability to identify and control specific experimental parameters in the design of the study. For example, a specific, well-characterised microorganism, the size and route of the infecting inoculum, the incubation time before treatment begins, and the dose, route, and duration of administration of the antimicrobial can all be controlled. The study end-points are typically quantitative and objective and may include rates of bacterial clearance, concentration of organisms in specific tissues or the proportion of animals with negative cultures after therapy. There is also the opportunity to compare multiple different treatment regimens under the same experimental conditions, including placebo treatment.

Experimental animal models also have a number of limitations; they are not a substitute for clinical trials but rather may provide preliminary data for the design and conduct of pivotal clinical trials. Because only one, or a few strains are studied, caution should be exercised extrapolating conclusions to other strains that may be implicated clinically. There are differences in the pharmacokinetics and pharmacodynamics of antimicrobials in small mammals. These differences may complicate the design or interpretation of experimental models. The studies are also technically demanding and require experience with these methods.

Animal models, with some notable exceptions, have a good track record in predicting efficacy of antimicrobials and have done especially well in predicting clinical failure. This review will highlight selected published data on the in-vivo activity of moxifloxacin in experimental animal models.

Results and Discussion

Two studies of moxifloxacin treatment of experimental meningitis have been reported. Schmidt and Dalhoff [1] investigated the treatment of meningitis due to a penicillin-susceptible pneumococcus using a rabbit model of experimental meningitis. An intracisternal catheter was placed for the inoculation of the pneumococcus and for obtaining repeated samples to measure drug concentrations and bacterial counts over time. Treatment with moxifloxacin began 12 h after direct intracisternal inoculation and consisted of a 5 mg/kg loading dose followed by an infusion of 2.5, 10 or 20 mg/kg/h for the 12 h treatment period. Dexamethasone in addition to moxifloxacin 10 mg/kg/h was also studied as was ceftriaxone 10 mg/kg/h.

The mean moxifloxacin concentrations in CSF ranged from approximately 30 to 50% of the concentration in serum (Table 1). Moxifloxacin treatment produced a dose-dependent decrease in the number of surviving bacteria (Table 2). The maximum rate of decrease was obtained with 10 mg/kg/h which reduced the surviving bacteria to approximately 10% of the original load in 3 h. At 10 mg/kg/h or greater, moxifloxacin was similar in activity to ceftriaxone. The addition of dexamethasone to moxifloxacin had no effect either on the penetration of moxifloxacin into CSF or on the rate of bacterial clearance. The release of lipoteichoic acid was also measured in this study and was more rapid in the animals treated with ceftriaxone than in animals treated with moxifloxacin.

Østergaard et al. [2] also reported results from an experimental meningitis model, using a penicillin-resistant pneumococcus strain (penicillin MIC 1 µg/mL). Rabbits were infected with a direct intracisternal inoculation of 10^6 cfu

Table 1. A comparison of the steady state concentrations of moxifloxacin or ceftriaxone in CSF and serum in an experimental model of pneumococcal meningitis in rabbits. Adapted from Schmidt [1]

Treatment	Mean Concentration (mg/L)	
	CSF	Serum
Moxifloxacin 2.5 mg/kg/h	1.9	3.3
Moxifloxacin 10 mg/kg/h	3.8	10.4
Moxifloxacin 10 mg/kg/h + dexamethasone 1 mg/kg/h	3.3	12.3
Moxifloxacin 20 mg/kg/h	8.5	19.8
Ceftriaxone 10 mg/kg/h	7.1	159.0

Table 2
The rate of decrease in the concentration of pneumocci in CSF of rabbits with experimental meningitis treated with moxifloxacin or ceftriaxone. Data from Schmidt [1]

Treatment	Mean $\Delta \log 10$ Cfu/mL/h	
Moxifloxacin 2.5 mg/kg/h	-0.19	
Moxifloxacin 10 mg/kg/h	-0.32	$(p < 0.05)$
Moxifloxacin 10 mg/kg/h + dexamethasone 1 mg/kg/h	-0.25	
Moxifloxacin 20 mg/kg/h	-0.31	
Ceftriaxone 10 mg/kg/h	-0.39	

of pneumococci. Treatment with moxifloxacin or vancomycin was begun 10 h later. Moxifloxacin and vancomycin were administered as two iv bolus doses 5 h apart; ceftriaxone was given as a single dose due to its long half-life. The study strain's MIC of ceftriaxone and vancomycin was 0.5 µg/mL and the moxifloxacin MIC was 0.125 µg/mL. The response to the treatments was monitored by culturing the CSF at 3, 5, 10 and 24 h.

Table 3 shows the results of pharmacokinetic studies in the CSF. The moxifloxacin C_{max} in CSF was approximately 80% of the serum C_{max}. Each treatment regimen was more effective than was no therapy (Fig. 1). Changing the moxifloxacin dose from two 20 mg/kg doses to either a single dose of 40 mg/kg or two doses of 40 mg/kg produced decreases in the bacterial concentration at 3 to 10 h post-treatment. However, at 24 h there was little difference in the concentration of surviving bacteria between the different dosing regimens. Moxifloxacin was as effective as vancomycin or ceftriaxone for this strain of penicillin-resistant pneumococcus.

The issues of multi-drug resistance among pneumococci and the activities of fluoroquinolones against pneumococci have been discussed extensively. Rouse et al. [3] compared in vivo the relative activities of moxifloxacin, ciprofloxacin, levofloxacin or sparfloxacin using an immunocompetent murine model of penicillin-resistant streptococcal pneumonia. A blunt tipped feeding tube was placed into the trachea and 10^6 cfu of *Streptococcus pneumoniae* was inoculated intratracheally. Four hours later, treatment with fluoroquinolones was begun and

Table 3. The pharmacokinetics of moxifloxacin, ceftriaxone and vancomycin in the CSF of rabbits with experimental pneumococcal meningitis. Data from Østergaard [2]

Treatment	CSF		
	C_{max}	AUC_{0-24h}	$T_{>MBC}$
Moxifloxacin 20 mg/kg[a]	6.3	34.9	22 h
Moxifloxacin 40 mg/kg[a]	8.3	62.4	24 h
Ceftriaxone 125 mg/kg	9.8	N/A	>24 h
Vancomycin 20 mg/kg[a]	2.6	N/A	>24 h

[a] Two doses, 5 h apart.

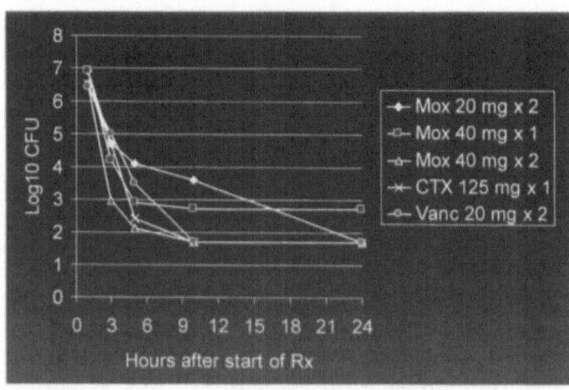

Fig. 1
Median concentrations of bacteria in CSF after the start of antibiotic therapy for experimental meningitis due to a penicillin-resistant pneumococcus strain. Mox = moxifloxacin, CTX = ceftriaxone, Vanc = vancomycin. See text for specific dosing regimens. Adapted from Østergaard [2]

consisted of 4 oral doses at 6 h intervals. The more frequent dosing schedule was chosen due to the shorter half-life of these antibiotics in mice compared to humans. The primary end-point was the number of surviving bacteria in lung tissue, expressed as log_{10} cfu/gram tissue. The pneumococcus strain used in vivo was chosen from a group of 27 penicillin-resistant clinical isolates. It had a MIC of penicillin of 2 µg/mL which was the median for the group. The MIC (µg/mL) of ciprofloxacin, levofloxacin, sparfloxacin and moxifloxacin were 2.0, 0.5, 0.25 and 0.125. The activity in vitro of the fluoroquinolones was unaffected by penicillin resistance.

The outcome of treatment with each fluoroquinolone was significantly better than no treatment (Table 4), as assessed by bacterial clearance from lung tissue. Moxifloxacin was significantly more effective than the other fluoroquinolones tested, resulting in 11 sterile mice in the group of 15 treated with moxifloxacin (Table 4). Although the peak concentration (Table 4) of moxifloxacin in serum was less than that of ciprofloxacin or levofloxacin, the AUC:MIC ratio favoured moxifloxacin due to its lower MIC.

Results of treatment of murine experimental hematogenously disseminated tuberculosis were reported by Ji et al. [4]. Mice were each given an intravenous inoculation of 10^6 cfu of *Mycobacterium tuberculosis* followed by 4 weeks treat-

Table 4. Results of treatment of experimental pneumococcal pneumonia in immunocompetent mice

Treatment	30'/60' Conc	#sterile/ #treated	Median log_{10} cfu
Placebo	–	0/17	8.1
Cipro 100 mg/kg	5.4/2.5	0/9	5.9
Levo 50 mg/kg	5.2/4.0	1/10	4.3
Spar 50 mg/kg	0.8/2.3	1/11	3.9
Moxi 100 mg/kg	2.0/1.3	11/15	0.5

Moxi p < 0.05, moxi vs. all others. Cipro – ciprofloxacin; Levo – levofloxacin; Spar – sparfloxacin; Moxi – moxifloxacin.

ment with isoniazid, moxifloxacin, sparfloxacin, or clinafloxacin. The MIC of each fluoroquinolone for the study strain was 0.5 μg/mL. The end-points were survival, bacterial concentration in the spleen and spleen weight. The treatment regimens were clinafloxacin, sparfloxacin or moxifloxacin given 6 times/week at 25, 50 or 100 mg/kg; isoniazid 25 mg/kg six times/week was the positive control. Due to the interest in directly observed therapy, sparfloxacin was also administered 100 mg/kg once/week.

After 28 days there was 50% mortality in both the untreated controls and in the clinafloxacin treated mice. Isoniazid, each of the sparfloxacin doses, including the once weekly dose, and each of the moxifloxacin doses was effective in preventing mortality. The bacterial concentration in spleen tissue at the beginning of the study and on day 30 is illustrated in Fig. 2. In the untreated animals and in the clinafloxacin treated mice there was a 10-fold increase in bacteria in the spleen during 30 days. Thus, clinafloxacin was ineffective even though it was active in vitro. Treatment with isoniazid produced a 4 to 5 log reduction in the bacteria in the spleen. Sparfloxacin and moxifloxacin were also effective and caused a dose dependent decrease in bacterial concentration. Isoniazid, sparfloxacin or moxifloxacin showed similar efficacy as measured by survival and by dose dependent reductions in bacteria in the spleen. On a weight basis, moxifloxacin was more potent than sparfloxacin in reducing bacterial load.

Endocarditis is often considered among the most stringent tests of bactericidal antimicrobial activity because of the ineffectiveness of the host immune system in this model. Successful treatment depends directly on the bactericidal activity of the antimicrobial agent in a lesion which is difficult for antimicrobials to penetrate, against microorganisms which are in a slowed metabolic state. Entenza et al. [5] used a rat model of infective endocarditis to compare treatment with moxifloxacin to treatment with ciprofloxacin or vancomycin for 3 different strains of MRSA. Two strains were susceptible and one was resistant to ciprofloxacin; all three strains were susceptible to moxifloxacin. The MIC values (μg/mL) for the susceptible strains were 0.25 and 0.12 for ciprofloxacin and moxifloxacin, respectively; for the resistant strains they were 8 and 0.25, respec-

Fig. 2
The effect of antibiotics on the mean number of *M. tuberculosis* organisms in spleens of mice. Error bars represent standard deviations. CNX = clinafloxacin, MXFX= moxifloxacin, SPFX = sparfloxacin, INH = isoniazid. Dosing regimens are described in text. Reprinted with permission from Ji [4]

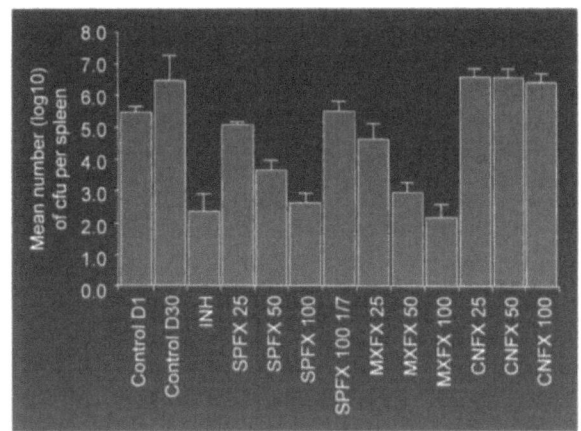

Table 5. The outcome of treatment with moxifloxacin, ciprofloxacin or vancomycin in experimental endocarditis in rats infected with either ciprofloxacin-sensitive (Cipro-S) or ciprofloxacin-resistant (Cipro-R) strains of MRSA. [5]

Strain	No. of infected animals/Total			
	No Rx	Moxi	Cipro	Vanc
Cip-S #1	6/6	1/11	3/8	5/11
Cip-S #2	6/6	0/12[a]	3/8	3/8
Cip-R	8/8	1/12[b]	5/5	3/9

[a] p = 0.05, moxi vs cipro or vanc.
[b] p = 0.001, moxi vs cipro.

tively. Antimicrobial treatment was continued for 3 days and the doses were chosen so that the concentration in rat serum closely matched the expected human serum levels produced by doses of ciprofloxacin 750 mg bid, moxifloxacin 400 mg qd, or vancomycin 1 g bid. The end point was the number of non-sterile animals at the end of therapy.

There was no statistically significant difference in outcome (Table 5) between the different treatments with one of the ciprofloxacin-susceptible strains. Moxifloxacin produced a significantly better outcome than ciprofloxacin or vancomycin with the second ciprofloxacin-susceptible strain. With the ciprofloxacin-resistant strain, ciprofloxacin failed in 5 of 5 rats, vancomycin failed in 3 of 9 rats, while moxifloxacin produced a successful outcome in 11 of 12 rats. Had rats not been sacrificed and allowed to survive without further treatment, it is possible some in the moxifloxacin-treated group may not have been free of infection. Nevertheless, this study provided evidence that some staphylococci resistant to one fluoroquinolone may still be effectively treated with another.

Conclusion

Moxifloxacin has been shown to be effective in animal models of meningitis, penicillin-resistant pneumococcal pneumonia, tuberculosis and endocarditis. Its activity against ciprofloxacin-resistant MRSA in the endocarditis model indicated that cross-resistance may not be universal among fluoroquinolones. The results of these studies suggest that moxifloxacin may have clinical efficacy in treating a range of infectious disease.

References

1. Schmidt H, Dalhoff A, Stuertz K, Trostdorf F, Chen V, Schneider O et al. (1998) Moxifloxacin in the therapy of experimental pneumococcal meningitis. Antimicrobial Agents and Chemotherapy 42:1397–1401
2. Østergaard C, Sørensen TK, Knudsen JD, Frimot-Møller N (1998) Evaluation of moxifloxacin, a new 8-methoxyquinolone, for treatment of meningitis caused by a penicillin-resistant pneumococcus in rabbits. Antimicrobial Agents and Chemotherapy 42:1706–1712

3. Rouse MS, Piper KE, Patel R, Wilson WR, Steckelberg JM (1997) In vitro and in vivo activity of ciprofloxacin, levofloxacin, sparfloxacin or moxifloxacin against penicillin-resistant Streptococcus pneumoniae. In: Programme and Abstracts of the Seventh Interscience Conference on Antimicrobial Agents and Chemotherapy, Toronto, 1997, Abstract B3

4. Ji B, Lounis N, Maslo C, Triffot-Pernot C, Bonnafous J, Gosset J (1998) In vivo and in vitro activities of moxifloxacin and clinafloxacin against *Mycobacterium tuberculosis.* Antimicrobial Agents and Chemotherapy 42:2066–2069

5. Entenza JM, Giddey M, Glauser MP, Moreillon P (1998) Efficacy of the Novel Quinolone BAY 12-8039 (Moxifloxacin) in the Treatment of Experimental Endocarditis (EE) Due to Ciprofloxacin-Susceptible (CIP-S) and Ciprofloxacin-Resistant (CIP-R), Methicillin-Resistant Staphylococcus aureus (MRSA). In: Programme and Abstracts of the International Congress of Antimicrobial Agents and Chemotherapy, San Diego, 1998, Abstract B-78

CHAPTER 21

Current Thinking About Pharmacokinetics and Pharmacodynamics of Antimicrobials

JOHN TURNIDGE

Abstract. In-vitro observations show that concentration-dependent killing is an important feature of fluoroquinolones. They have a moderate post-antibiotic effect and for some bacteria they have the propensity to select resistant mutants; the in-vitro modeling has demonstrated that the most problematic organism is *Pseudomonas spp.* and perhaps *Staphylococcus aureus.* These are organisms whose MIC values are close to the breakpoints.

There have been many studies that confirm the concept of the AUC/MIC ratio and C_{max}/ MIC ratio and virtually eliminated time above MIC as a predictor of efficacy. Optimal bactericidal effect requires the AUC/MIC ratio to be greater than 100. Selection of resistant mutants is unlikely with a C_{max}/MIC ratio greater than 10 [1–3]. There are three published clinical studies [4–6] demonstrating that these parameters are predictors of efficacy.

This chapter will discuss pharmacodynamic concepts and how the information can be used in a practical way and where this information might lead in the future.

One of the significant uses of the AUC/MIC ratio is the ability to make comparisons between drugs. Most animal models have indicated that a ratio AUC/MIC of 100 or more was required for successful anti-infective treatment. Importantly, small changes in the AUC will not be as significant as one to two fold dilutions in the MIC value. The same applies to the C_{max}/MIC ratios.

The AUC/MIC ratios were calculated for several fluoroquinolones using published data for MIC values (Table 1) and pharmacokinetic data (Table 2) for the recommended doses for each drug. The pharmacokinetic data were at steady state. There are also data (Table 2) on protein binding, because this is now potentially an issue. Although there is reasonable evidence that it is important for beta-lactams, it is not known if it is an issue with the fluoroquinolones. The

Table 1
The MIC_{90} values for fluoro-quinolones against *S. aureus* and *S. pneumoniae*

Fluoroquinolone	MIC_{90} (µg/mL)	
	S. aureus	S. pneumoniae
Ciprofloxacin	0.5	2
Grepafloxacin	0.1	0.39
Levofloxacin	0.4	1.56
Moxifloxacin	0.06	0.12–0.25
Sparfloxacin	0.125	0.5
Trovafloxacin	0.06	0.12–0.25

Table 2. The pharmacokinetics of fluoroquinolones after administration of the clinically recommended dose

Agent	Dose	C_{max}	AUC_{0-24}	PB %
Sparfloxacin	400 mg to 200 mg qd	0.6	16.4	45
Levofloxacin	500 mg daily	5.2	61.1	24–38
Grepafloxacin	400 mg daily	0.9	11.4	50
Grepafloxacin	600 mg daily	1.4	19.7	50
Trovafloxacin	200 mg daily	2.2	30.4	70
Moxifloxacin	400 mg daily	4.5	48.0	30–45

PB% – percentage protein binding.

Fig. 1
Comparison of the AUC/MIC
ratios for fluoroquinolones
against *S. aureus*

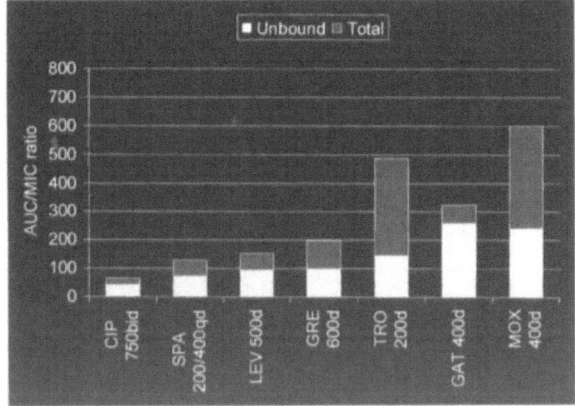

AUC/MIC ratios for fluoroquinolones against *S. aureus* are displayed in Fig. 1 where it is possible to compare their potential efficacy. If optimal bactericidal effect requires a ratio AUC/MIC of 100, then six of the seven drugs shown would be effective against *S. aureus*.

Clearly, a drug with a low MIC value and a large AUC would compare favourably against others that had either a high MIC or a small AUC. The ratios plotted in Fig. 1 indicated moxifloxacin was the most potent of the group against *S. aureus* with an AUC/MIC ratio of 800. Is there any value to having the ratio significantly greater than 100, or does this indicate wasted drug? There is opinion that ratios above 100, to some undefined maximum, are useful because it causes more rapid elimination of the organism.

Similar calculations for AUC/MIC ratios were made for *S. pneumoniae* and the data are illustrated in Fig. 2. These results showed that only two fluoroquinolones had an AUC/MIC ratio greater than 100, with moxifloxacin the greater. There have been proposals that an AUC/MIC ratio as low as 35 would still indicate efficacy. However, clinical studies have shown that AUC/MIC ratios of 100 or more provide maximal efficacy and will virtually guarantee cures in patients, and will decrease the development of resistance.

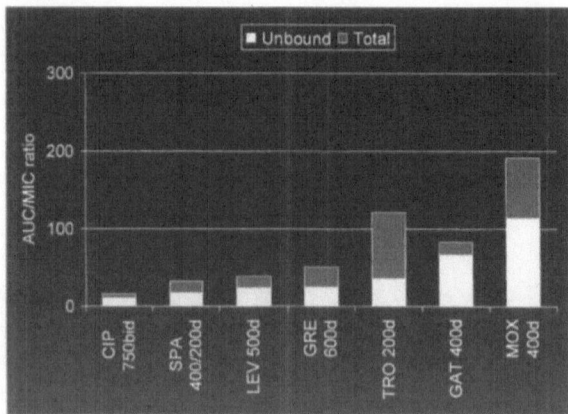

Fig. 2
Comparison of the AUC/MIC
ratios for fluoroquinolones
against *S. pneumoniae*

Table 3. Comparison of theoretical breakpoints based on AUC/MIC ratios with NCCLS listed breakpoints for quinolones

Fluoroquinolone	Regimen	Breakpoint (μu/mL)	
		PK/PD	NCCLS
Ciprofloxacin	500 mg bid	0.5	1
Ciprofloxacin	750 mg bid	0.5	1
Grepafloxacin	400 mg daily	0.125	1
Grepafloxacin	600 mg daily	0.25	1
Levofloxacin	500 mg daily	1	2
Moxifloxacin	400 mg daily	0.5	–
Sparfloxacin	400 mg to 200 mg qd	0.25	0.25–0.5
Trovafloxacin	200 mg daily	0.5	1

By assuming an optimal AUC/MIC ratio of 100, and taking the pharmaco-kinetic data from Table 2, it is possible to calculate the theoretical breakpoints for the MIC values. These are shown in Table 3 where they are compared to the NCCLS breakpoints. For each fluoroquinolone the calculated breakpoint was lower than the current accepted value. This is an important issue for future consideration.

Finally, a comment about the concept of selecting for resistant mutants. What is the appropriate AUC, is it based on the first dose or is it at steady state? It would be preferable to obtain it as early as possible in treatment, especially for the sub-optimal drugs. Treating respiratory pathogens such as *S. pneumoniae* with sub-optimal AUC/MIC ratios will select resistant mutants and may jeopardise the drugs that give optimal ratios. Furthermore, consideration should be given to measuring plasma levels in problematic patients so that there is confidence that appropriate drug doses are given that provide AUC/MIC ratios above 100.

References

1. Drusano GL, Johnson D, Rosen M, Standiford MC (1993) Pharmacodynamics of a fluoro-quinolone antimicrobial agent in a neutropenic rat model of Pseudomonas sepsis. Antimicrob Agents Chemother 37:483–490
2. Craig WA (1998) Pharmacokinetic/pharmacodynamic parameters: rationale for antibacterial dosing of mice and men. Clin Infect Dis 26:1–12
3. Watanabe Y, Ebert S, Craig WA (1992) AUC/MIC ratio is unifying parameter for comparison on in-vivo activity among fluoroquinolones. In: Program and Abstracts of the 32nd Interscience Conference on Antimicrobial Agents and Chemotherapy, Anaheim, p117 [Abstract number 42]
4. Forrest A, Nix DE, Ballow CH, Goss TF, Birmingham MC, Schentag JJ (1993) Pharmacodynamics of intravenous ciprofloxacin in seriously ill patients. Antimicrob Agents Chemother 37:1073–1081
5. Preston SL, Drusano GL, Berman AL, Fowler CL, Chow AT, Dornseif B, Reichl V, Natarajan J, Corrado M (1998) Pharmacodynamics of levofloxacin. A new paradigm for early clinical trials. JAMA 279:125–129
6. Forrest A, Chodosh S, Amantea MA, Collins DA, Schentag JJ (1997) Pharmacokinetics and pharmacodynamics of oral grepafloxacin in patients with acute exacerbations of chronic bronchitis. J Antimicrob Chemother 40 (Suppl. A):45–57

Pharmacology of Moxifloxacin – Absorption, Distribution, Metabolism and Excretion

CARL ERIK NORD

Abstract. In humans, moxifloxacin is rapidly absorbed, the bioavailability is high (approx. 90%) and the plasma half-life is between 11.4–15.2 h depending on the dose given, indicating a once-daily treatment regimen. There is good distribution to saliva, interstitial fluids and lung tissues. The main metabolites are N-sulphate (M1) and acylglucuronide (M2). Phase II metabolism occurs in humans but no P450 metabolism. No antimicrobial activity of M1 and M2 is observed. Moxifloxacin is eliminated via metabolic, renal and biliary/faecal routes. About 22% of a moxifloxacin dose is excreted via the kidneys as unmetabolised moxifloxacin, while 14% and 2.5% of a dose is renally excreted as acylglucuronide (M2) and N-sulphate (M1), respectively. Recovery in faeces was 26% for unmetabolised moxifloxacin and 35% for N-sulphate (M1). Moxifloxacin has a good pharmacokinetic profile for treatment of respiratory tract infections.

Introduction

The development of moxifloxacin was the result of a process planned to produce a molecule with well defined antimicrobial properties. The pharmacokinetic studies in animals showed that it was well absorbed in mice, rats, monkeys, dogs and minipigs reaching acceptable C_{max} and AUC value and with a moderate to long half life. It was shown to accumulate in rat lung tissue following both oral and intravenous administration. This provided a good basis to investigate pharmacokinetics in humans.

Results and Discussion

When moxifloxacin was given as a single dose, either orally or intravenously, there was good absorption and good bioavailability (approximately 90%). The data [1–3] in Table 1 show the linear relationship between dose administered, C_{max} and AUC. The data also show that the plasma half life was about 12 h. The pharmacokinetic properties were also good following treatment for 8 days. For example, a once daily dose of 400 mg produced a C_{max} of 3.2 μg/mL, an AUC of 33.9 μg.h/mL and a $T_{1/2}$ of 15.2 h. A comparison of a single dose of 400 mg given either iv or po showed almost identical plasma concentration time curves, with an expected higher value for C_{max} following iv administration. The saliva concentrations of moxifloxacin were slightly higher than plasma. For example, a single administration of 400 mg moxifloxacin po resulted in a C_{max} of 6.3 μg/mL and an AUC of 40.9 μg.h/mL in saliva; the $T_{1/2}$ was similar to plasma at about

Table 1. The absorption and bioavailability in humans after single doses of moxifloxacin

Dose (mg)	Route	C_{max} (mg/L)	AUC (mg.h/L)	V/F_{SS} (L/kg)	$T_{1/2}$ (h)	CL_R (L/h)
100	Intravenous	1.2	8.9	2.0	13.0	2.2
200	Intravenous	2.1	17.9	1.9	12.7	2.2
400	Intravenous	4.6	36.9	1.8	13.4	2.8
50	Oral	0.3	3.9	2.5	11.4	2.8
100	Oral	0.6	8.5	2.9	12.2	2.4
200	Oral	1.2	15.4	3.3	14.0	2.6
400	Oral	2.5	26.9	3.6	13.1	3.0
600	Oral	3.2	39.9	3.3	12.5	2.7
800	Oral	4.7	59.9	2.8	12.3	2.5

12 h. The high moxifloxacin concentrations in saliva indicate it may be useful to eradicate pathogens in the oropharynx.

Several studies have measured the penetration of fluoroquinolones into lung tissue. Data[4] from these studies, Table 2, show that moxifloxacin had favourable penetration compared to the other quinolones. These data suggest its potential usefulness in the treatment of respiratory tract infections. When one compares the plasma and lung tissue concentrations of the fluoroquinolones with their MIC values against respiratory tract bacterial pathogens, it is clear from the data[4] in Table 3 that they are more than adequate to treat respiratory infections. The data also show the favourable properties of moxifloxacin compared to trovafloxacin and levofloxacin.

Moxifloxacin yielded two metabolites [3], a sulfo-compound and an acyl-glucuronide, neither of which had antimicrobial activity. Their structures in relation to the parent molecule and their excretion in urine and faeces are illustrated in Fig. 1. Active moxifloxacin was found in both urine and faeces. There is no cytochrome P_{450} mediated metabolism of moxifloxacin, so only phase 2 metabolism is relevant in humans. As the two metabolites were inactive, the measurement of tissue concentrations by bioassay were amounts of the parent molecule. The renal excretion profiles of moxifloxacin and the two metabolites are shown [3] in Fig. 2. Administration by either the po or the iv route produced the same excretion profiles. The plasma concentration time curves for the two metabolites are shown

Table 2. The concentration of fluoroquinolones in human lung tissue

Fluoroquinolone	Dose (mg)	Serum C_{max} (mg/L)	Bronchial mucosa (mg/kg)	Epithelial lining fluid (mg/L)	Alveolar Macrophages (mg/L)
Moxifloxacin	400	3.3	5.5	24.4	113.6
Trovafloxacin	200	1.4	1.5	4.0	19.1
Sparfloxacin	400	0.5	1.3	5.8	9.6
Grepafloxacin	600	1.8	5.3	27.1	27.6

Table 3 a. Plasma and lung tissue concentrations of fluoroquinolones

Antibiotic	Oral dose (mg)		Plasma (mg/L)	Bronchial mucosa (mg/kg)	Epithelial lining fluid (mg/L)	Alveolar macrophage (mg/L)
Moxifloxacin	400	Peak	2.5–5.0	5.5	24.4	113.6
		Trough	0.5	1.0	3.5	38.6
Trovafloxacin	200	Peak	1.4–2.2	1.5	4.0	19.1
		Trough	0.4	ND	0..9	10.2
Levofloxacin	500	Peak	6.6	8.3	10.9	41.9
		Trough	1.2	ND	ND	13.9

Table 3 b. MIC values (µg/mL) of fluoroquinolones against respiratory tract pathogens

Antibiotic	MIC (mµ/mL)		
	S. pneumoniae	H. influenzae	M. catarrhalis
Moxifloxacin	0.125–0.5	0.031–0.063	0.125
Trovafloxacin	0.12–0.25	0.01–0.05	0.03
Levofloxacin	1-2	0.015–0.031	0.06–0.0125

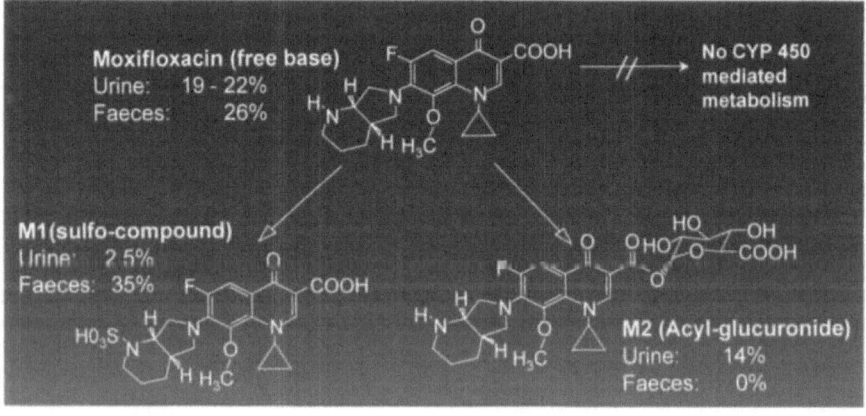

Fig. 1. The metabolism of moxifloxacin in humans following a single dose, showing the recovery in urine and faeces

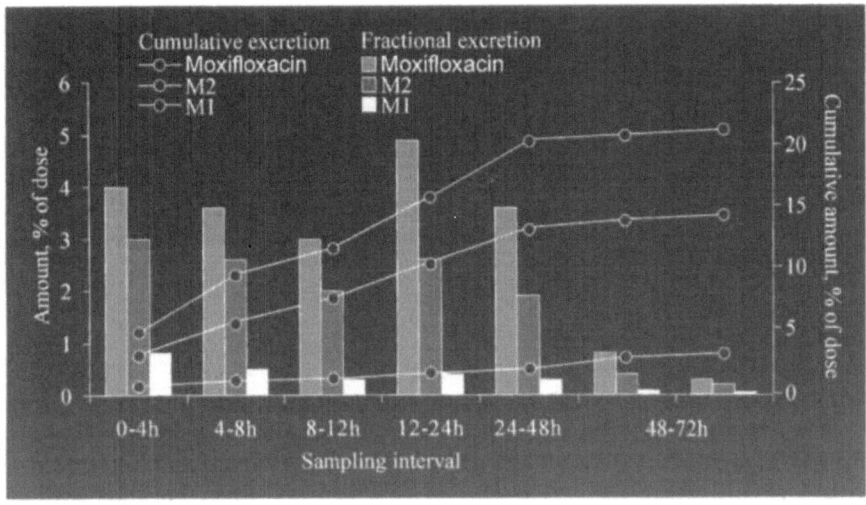

Fig. 2 The renal excretion of moxifloxacin and its metabolites following a single po doses of 400 mg. Bars = fractional excretion; lines = cumulative excretion; n = 6

Fig. 3
The geometric mean plasma concentration time curves of moxifloxacin metabolites. M1 (sulfocompound) and M2 (glucuronide) following a single 400 mg dose of moxifloxacin (n = 8)

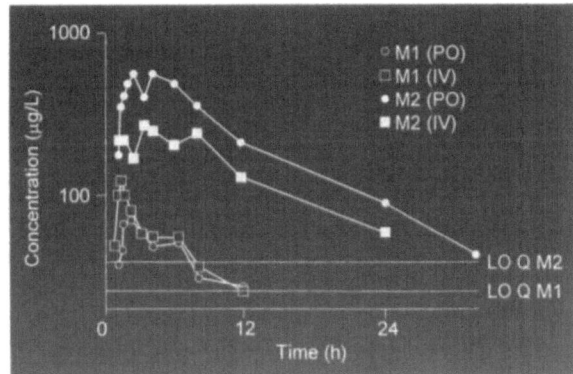

in Fig. 3. As expected, the plasma concentration of the sulfo-metabolite was low compared to the concentration of the glucuronide-metabolite.

The metabolic profile of moxifloxacin contributed to the safe use of the drug in patients. The absence of metabolism via the cytochrome P_{450} route contributed to its lack of significant drug interactions. Its balanced excretion via renal, faecal and metabolic pathways minimised the risk of its accumulating in high risk patients, e.g. those with renal on hepatic impairment. It is interesting to compare the excretion patterns (Fig. 4) of moxifloxacin to those of other fluoroquinolones. This balance suggests that no dosage adjustments will be needed, thus providing convenience to the profile of the drug.

Fig. 4
The comparison of excretion
patterns of fluoroquinolones
Moxi – moxifloxacin;
Trova – trovafloxacin;
Levo – levofloxacin;
Grepa – grepafloxacin;
Spar – sparfloxacin

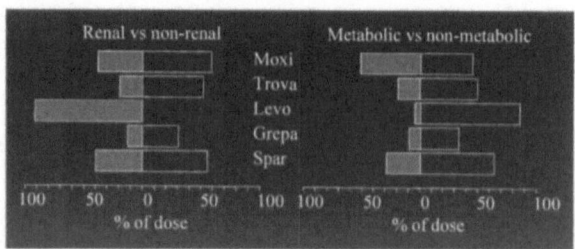

Conclusion

Moxifloxacin has several of the characteristics for the treatment of community respiratory tract infections. In addition to MIC of the values of the main pathogens which are exceeded over a 24 hour period by both serum and tissue concentrations, moxifloxacin has a balanced metabolism and excretion and is free of most strong interactions except the classical quinolone cation interaction.

References

1. Stass H, Dalhoff A, Kubitza D, Schuhly U (1998) Pharmacokinetics, safety, and tolerability of ascending single doses of moxifloxacin, a new 8-methoxy quinolone, administered to healthy subjects. Antimicrobial Agents and Chemotherapy 42:2060–2065
2. Stass H, Kubitza D (1998) Cross over study to assess the absolute bioavailability and absorption characteristics of BAY 12-8039. In: Programme and Abstracts of the Eight International Conference of Infectious Diseases, Boston, MA
3. Stass H, Delesen H, Kubitza D (1998) Determination of excretion patterns of BAY 12-8039 following single oral and intravenous doses. In: Programme and Abstracts of the Eight International Conference on Infectious Diseases, Boston, MA
4. Andrews J, Honeybourne D, Jevons G, Wise R (1998) Penetration of moxifloxacin into bronchial mucosa, epithelial lining fluid and alveolar macrophages following a single 400 mg oral dose. In: International Congress of Antimicrobial Agents and Chemotherapy, Abstract A29

CHAPTER 23

Antimicrobial Drug-Drug Interactions – Focus on Fluoroquinolones

23

GARY E. STEIN

Abstract. Clinically significant drug-drug interactions can occur with all classes of antimicrobial agents. Although the fluoroquinolones are a relatively safe group of compounds, some agents have been associated with clinically significant pharmacokinetic and pharmacodynamic drug interactions. Pharmacokinetic interactions include diminished absorption due to antacids or opiates, alteration in theophylline metabolism and a decrease in fluoroquinolone excretion due to concomitant probenecid. Pharmacodynamic effects have been observed with cyclosporine, warfarin and fenbufen. Moxifloxacin is a new fluoroquinolone that does not alter the pharmacokinetics of other drugs (e.g. theophylline, warfarin, digoxin) and is unlikely to provoke harmful pharmacodynamic drug interactions. With the exception of diminished absorption due to certain divalent cations, moxifloxacin appears to lack significant drug-drug interactions.

Introduction

The characteristic requirement for drugs is that they are not only efficacious, but also safe. An important component of a safety profile is a lack of significant drug interactions. All classes of antibiotics have potential drug-drug interactions which require awareness and appropriate clinical management. There are well known drug interactions that lead to changes in the absorption of antibiotics. Examples are the chelation effect with tetracycline and iron or calcium that reduces absorption. Similar reduction of ketoconazole absorption occurs when cimetidine is given to reduce stomach acidity. Interactions between erythromycin and theophylline lead to decreased metabolism and elevated plasma levels of theophylline that can lead to seizures. There are beneficial interactions, such as combining probenecid with ampicillin to slow the excretion and prolong the effective half-life of the antibiotic to improve its efficacy as a treatment for gonococcal infections.

There are also well known pharmacodynamic interactions. For example, the cephalosporin, cefotetan, can enhance the vitamin K-dependent clotting effect of warfarin. There are interactions between aminoglycosides and skeletal muscle relaxants that can cause respiratory depression. Other drug combinations, such as ampicillin and allopurinol, increase the risk of rashes in patients. Some of the same types of drug interactions are seen with the fluoroquinolones. This review will focus on pharmacokinetic and pharmacodynamic drug interactions of the fluoroquinolones, with an emphasis on moxifloxacin.

Results and Discussion

Clinical experience during the last decade has shown that the fluoroquinolones, as a class, have diminished absorption when administered with multivalent metal cations, such as aluminium, magnesium, zinc, iron and calcium. The fluoroquinolones form an unabsorbable complex with the metal cation decreasing absorption as much as 90%. Either they should not be administered concomitantly or the medications should be taken at different times. Antacids (Maalox) and iron supplements decreased the absorption of moxifloxacin reducing the maximum plasma concentration (C_{max}) by 80% and the area under the plasma concentration curve (AUC) by about 40%. The bioavailability was not significantly altered when moxifloxacin was administered 2 h before or 4 h after Maalox [1, 2].

Drugs which affect gut motility also have an effect on absorption. Concomitant administration of intravenous morphine with trovafloxacin reduced its AUC by 36%. Opiates, alone or in combination with anticholinergics, reduced by 50% the C_{max} and AUC of ciprofloxacin given orally to surgical patients [3]. There is a suggestion that this may not be a class effect for all fluoroquinolones and a study with moxifloxacin is in progress.

Several fluoroquinolones interact with the 1A2 isoenzyme of the cytochrome P_{450} complex, leading to decreased metabolism of R-warfarin, theophylline, caffeine and benzodiazepines. The fluoroquinolones implicated in these reactions include ciprofloxacin, norfloxacin and enoxacin. These drug interactions can be clinically significant; for example ciprofloxacin and theophylline can result in nausea/vomiting and seizures. With the exception of grepafloxacin, whose potential for metabolic interaction is similar to ciprofloxacin, the newer fluoroquinolones do not alter theophylline metabolism.

Moxifloxacin has been shown to have no inhibitory effect on theophylline pharmacokinetics in healthy volunteers following either a single dose or steady state dosing. Consequently, it is expected that moxifloxacin will be a safe drug to use in combination with other widely used medications.

In general, the fluoroquinolones do not interact with the 2C9 isoenzyme of the cytochrome P_{450} complex and do not alter the pharmacokinetics of S-warfarin. However, increases in prothrombin time have been observed in many patients. This is probably due to a mechanism involving changes in the gut flora but does warrant continued monitoring. Moxifloxacin has been studied in healthy volunteers, where it was shown to have no effect on warfarin pharmacokinetics nor on clotting factors II, VII and X.

Fluoroquinolones, such as norfloxacin, ciprofloxacin and ofloxacin, which are mainly excreted via the renal tubules, can be affected by probenecid and cimetidine. Renal clearance can be reduced by about 30% by probenecid. There appears to be no clinical significance to the decreased renal clearance and this is probably due to a compensating increase in the metabolic clearance. Moxifloxacin is minimally (20%) excreted by the kidneys, so probenecid, as expected, exhibited no effect on plasma or urine pharmacokinetics in healthy volunteers.

There have been several cases of renal insufficiency in patients treated with ciprofloxacin and cyclosporine. Several studies have investigated the phenomenon, especially to determine if it is a pharmacokinetic interaction. No evidence for increased plasma cyclosporine levels was obtained to account for the decreased renal function. The precise mechanism remains undefined but it suggests that renal function be monitored when a fluoroquinolone is used with cyclosporine.

Sparfloxacin and grepafloxacin cause an increase in the electrocardiogram QTc interval. There is a potential for significant interactions with drugs that are used to treat ventricular tachycardia. There have been several reports of deaths when sparfloxacin was used with antiarrhythmia drugs, especially amiodarone. The recommendation is to avoid using these fluoroquinolones in patients who are being treated with antiarrhythmic drugs.

Conclusion

Moxifloxacin has the property to chelate with multivalent metal cations as do the other fluoroquinolones. This interaction leads to decreased absorption but can be avoided by staggering the doses of moxifloxacin and the other medication. Other drugs, e.g. cimetidine, do not affect absorption of moxifloxacin. There are no important metabolic interactions with theophylline, warfarin, digoxin and oral contraceptives. Furthermore there are no dramatic pharmacodynamic interactions detected with moxifloxacin. It would be prudent to continue to evaluate pharmacodynamic interactions with new broad-spectrum antibiotics.

References

1. Stass H, Kubitza D (1998) Moxifloxacin – Review of clinical pharmacokinetics interaction profile. In: Programme and Abstracts of the Sixth International Symposium on New Quinolones. Denver, CO
2. Stass H, Kern A (1998) Moxifloxacin – Review of clinical pharmacokinetics metabolism and excretion. In: Programme and Abstracts of the Sixth International Symposium on New Quinolones. Denver, CO
3. Morran C, McArdle C, Petitt L et al. (1989) Brief Report: Pharmacokinetics of orally administered ciprofloxacin in abdominal surgery. American Journal of Medicine 87 (Suppl 5A): 86S – 88S

Chapter 24

Pharmacology – Tissue Distribution 24

Ethan Rubinstein

Abstract. The fluoroquinolones are antibiotics with good pharmacokinetic and pharmaco-dynamic properties and broad spectrum of activity, resulting in excellent therapeutic results. Moxifloxacin penetrates well into most body tissues and fluids. It attains high levels in the various compartments of the pulmonary tract, including the alveolar lining fluid, the bronchial mucosa, and the alveolar macrophages. Penetration into CSF is approximately 40% and is not affected by co-administration of dexamethasone. These features make moxifloxacin a potentially valuable agent for a wide range of indications.

This review will focus specifically on moxifloxacin tissue distribution.

Moxifloxacin is highly bioavailable, so plasma concentrations following an oral dose are similar to those found after intravenous dosing. A comparison of iv and po moxifloxacin pharmacokinetics in humans following a 400 mg dose showed peak concentrations ranging between 3 and 5 μg/mL for both routes of administration. Moxifloxacin plasma half-life was approximately 11 h [1].

Saliva levels following a 400 mg po dose of moxifloxacin were comparable to those found in plasma and capillary blood (C_{max} of 3.63, 3.19 and 2.53 μg/mL, respectively), with lower concentrations found in subcutaneous tissue (C_{max} of 1.02 μg/mL). The half-life in plasma, saliva and capillary blood ranged from 11.9 to 14.3 h, while the rate of elimination from subcutaneous tissue was much more rapid (half-life of 2.5 h) [1].

Subcutaneous tissue, muscle, saliva and blister fluid concentrations of moxifloxacin were compared using a microdialysis model (see Fig. 1). Results showed

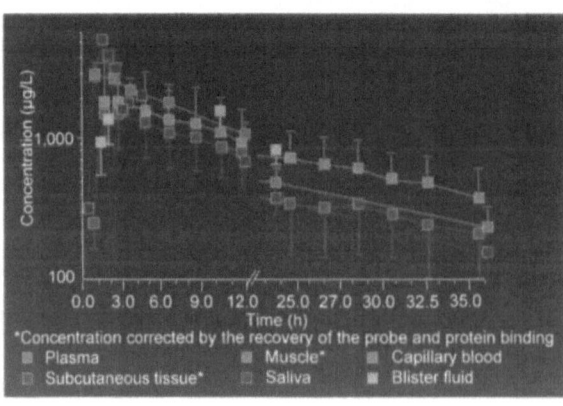

Fig. 1
The time course of plasma, subcutaneous tissue, muscle, saliva and blister fluid concentrations (geometric mean/SD) of moxifloxacin following a 400 mg iv dose

that moxifloxacin penetrated all these fluids in a similar manner, therefore plasma or serum concentrations should be indicative of penetration into other compartments. This relationship is further examined in Figs. 2–4 [1].

The time course for the ratio of concentration in skeletal muscle microdialysate versus plasma revealed that both the iv and po forms of moxifloxacin showed similar penetration. Ratios started around 0.2 and rose to 0.6 within 12 h of dosing. By 24 h post-dose, equilibrium was reached between plasma and muscle tissue and ratios were close to 1. For the subcutaneous transplant microdialysate, ratios versus plasma ranged from 3–4 over the first 12 h, reaching 6 around 36 h post-dose. Saliva pharmacokinetics were similar to those in plasma, and after rapid equilibrium, both routes of administration resulted in a site vs. plasma ratio between 0.9 and 1. Consequently, both iv and po moxifloxacin formulations may be equally useful in the eradication of meningococci in saliva.

Fig. 2
The time course of the geometric mean ratio of concentrations of moxifloxacin in skeletal muscle microdialysate vs. plasma

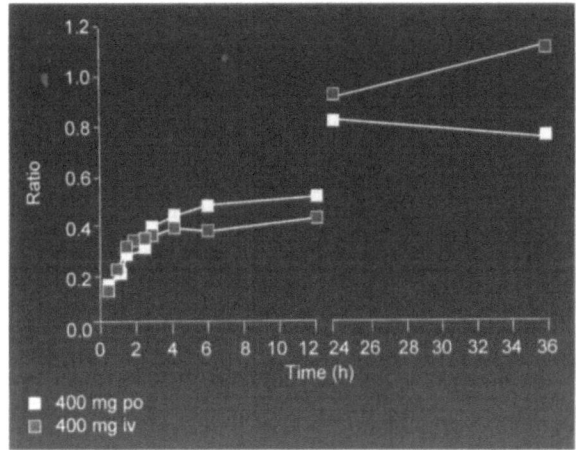

Fig. 3
The time course of the geometric mean ratio of concentrations of moxifloxacin in subcutaneous microdialysate vs. plasma

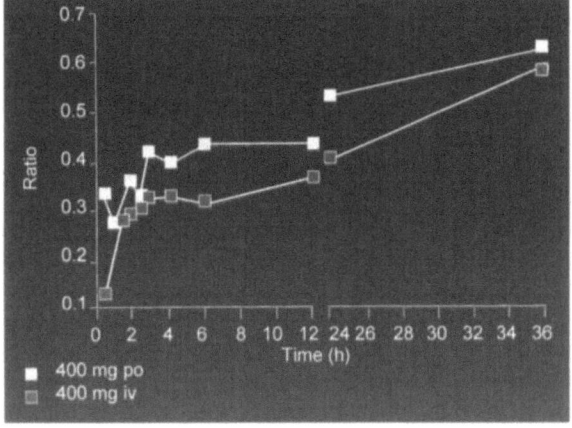

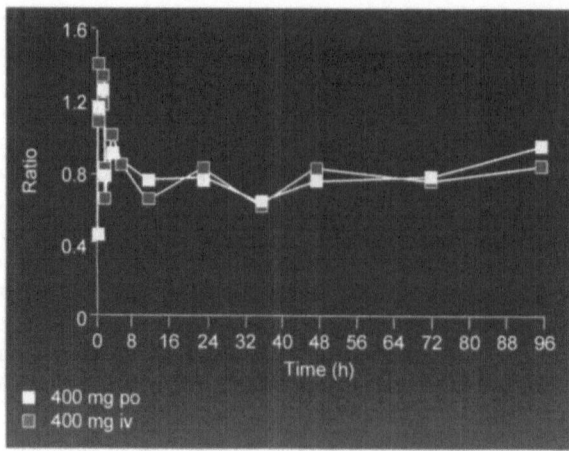

Fig. 4
The time course of the geometric mean ratio of concentrations of moxifloxacin in saliva vs. plasma

The penetration of moxifloxacin into human sinus mucosa was studied following multiple po dosings [2]. Mucosal concentration exceeded plasma concentration at all sampling times, with a sinus mucosa vs. plasma ratio of 2 over the first 6 h, increasing to approximately 4 at 36 h post-dose. Thus, soon after dosing there was favourable penetration of moxifloxacin into the sinus mucosa, suggesting that moxifloxacin would be useful in the treatment of bacterial sinusitis.

Moxifloxacin is primarily intended for treatment of lower respiratory tract infections, therefore concentrations in the bronchial mucosa (BM), in the epithelial lining fluid (ELF) and in alveolar macrophages (AM) are important. High concentrations of the drug were found in alveolar macrophages and in the epithelial lining fluid for 3, 12 and 24 h after drug administration. Site vs. plasma ratios ranged from 1.7 to 2 for BM, 6.6–7.4 for ELF and 18.8–89.4 for AM [3]. Based on experience with other fluoroquinolones, these results indicate that moxifloxacin can be successfully for the treatment of respiratory infections.

Moxifloxacin penetration into inflammatory interstitial (blister) fluid was investigated after po and iv dosing. The C_{max} values for both routes of administration were relatively high, about 60% of the corresponding plasma peak, with a t_{max} delayed by 1 to 2 h versus that of plasma. The extent of blister penetration was 83% for po and 93% for iv routes of administration [3].

The time course of blister fluid penetration showed that the blister fluid vs. plasma ratio for moxifloxacin was about 1.5 after 24 h. The ratio was lower in the early hours because it took some time to balance the concentration between blister fluid and the plasma compartments [1].

Streptococcus pneumoniae meningitis is an important complication of pneumococcal disease, and so it is also important to determine the extent of moxifloxacin penetration into cerebrospinal fluid (CSF). Using a rabbit meningitis model, data showed that CSF levels of moxifloxacin after 2.5, 5 and 10 mg doses were higher than most MIC values. The ratio of the penetration between CSF and serum was around 0.4 and dosing with 10 mg dexamethasone did not reduce the CSF penetration of moxifloxacin as it did for vancomycin and ceftriaxone [4].

These results are supported by another study which showed that moxifloxacin bactericidal activity against *S. pneumoniae* was not significantly different when administered with dexamethasone, and activity was comparable to that of ceftriaxone when administered alone [5].

Biliary moxifloxacin concentrations were examined in rabbits administered 15 mg/kg doses of moxifloxacin. As soon as 45 minutes after iv dosing, moxifloxacin concentrations in bile begin to greatly exceed plasma concentrations. This rise corresponds to the secretion of unmetabolised moxifloxacin into the gastrointestinal tract [6].

Moxifloxacin elimination is very low in the caecum and it is higher in the jejunum and ileum. Altogether about 7 to 8% of an iv administered dose is eliminated trans-epithelially via the gastrointestinal tract. This trans-epithelial elimination is an alternative pathway to the renal elimination, and if kidney function were blocked, it could account for up to 30 or 40% of the administered dose [7].

Conclusion

Moxifloxacin shows good penetration into most tissue compartments particularly those relevant to upper respiratory tract infections. Penetration into CSF is approximately 40% and is not affected by co-administration with dexamethasone. Moxifloxacin is actively secreted into the bile and approximately 7–8% of the dose is eliminated trans-epithelially.

References

1. Stass H, Brunner M, Eichler HG, Moller J-G, Muller M (1998) Comparison of skin blister fluid and interstitial tissue kinetics of moxifloxacin in healthy volunteers using microdialysis. Abstract A12 in Programme and Abstracts of the Eight International Conference of Infectious Diseases, Boston, MA
2. Gehanno P et al. (1999) Penetration of moxifloxacin (MXF) into sinus tissues following multiple oral dosings. Abstract 0201 in Programme and Abstracts of the 9th European Conference of Clinical Microbiology and Infectious Diseases (ECCMID), Berlin, Germany
3. Andrews J, Honeybourne G, Jevons G, Wise R (1998) Penetration of moxifloxacin into bronchial mucosa, epithelial lining fluid and alveolar macrophages following a single, 400-mg oral dose. Abstract A29 in Programme and Abstracts of the Eight International Conference of Infectious Diseases, Boston, MA
4. Schmidt H, Dalhof A, Stuertz K, Trostdorf F, Chen V, Scheider O et al. (1998) Moxifloxacin therapy of experimental pneumococcal meningitis. Antimicrobial Agents and Chemotherapy 42:1397–1401
5. Schmidt H, Dalhof A, Stuertz K, Trostdorf F, Kohlsdorfer C, Nau R (1998) Bay 12-8039 for experimental pneumococcal meningitis. In: Programme and Abstracts of the Eight International Conference of Infectious Diseases, Boston, MA
6. Rubinstein E, Masafiji A, Stehlman Y, Barziki A, Seger S (1998) Transepithelial intestinal elimination of moxifloxacin in rabbits. Abstract 122 in Programme and Abstracts of the International Congress of Antimicrobial Agents and Chemotherapy

CHAPTER 25

Fluoroquinolone Phototoxicity – Moxifloxacin in Context

25

JAMES FERGUSON

Abstract. Moxifloxacin is an 8-methoxy quinolone. This structure is believed to confer reduced phototoxicity. Moxifloxacin was investigated in 32 healthy human male volunteers using a randomised, double-blind placebo and positive control (lomefloxacin) phototest study.

Baseline and on-drug photosensitivity was determined across the ultraviolet/visible wavebands using a differentiation grating monochrometer. Placebo and moxifloxacin (200 or 400 mg/day) regimen failed to demonstrate phototoxicity. Lomefloxacin (400 mg/day) revealed significant UVA (335–365 ± 30 nm) dependent phototoxicity with a phototoxic index of 3–4. This effect rapidly normalised within 48 hours of stopping the drug. No photoprotective measures appear necessary while taking moxifloxacin (200 or 400 mg/day).

Introduction

Many drugs can induce photosensitization. The effects may be systemic or confined to the skin. The acute effects are not only unpleasant but can require hospitalisation of the patient. There are many mechanisms whereby drugs cause photosensitivity in the skin. The phototoxicity associated with each family of drugs has its own clinical features and timing. The symptoms of potential drug-induced phototoxicity in skin need to be differentiated from other possible dermatological problems.

What is drug phototoxicity? It is a non-immunological mediated skin reaction which can arise in any individual provided there is enough drug and exposure to appropriate irradiation. The irradiation is usually, but not always, UVA wavelengths (320–400 nm). This form of irradiation is present year round, it penetrates window glass, thin clothing and water; it increases with reflection and altitude and is reasonably well absorbed by modern sunscreens.

There is a wide range of reports of phototoxicity of fluoroquinolones; the incidence varies from 0–20% even with the same drug. The clinical features are painful erythema progressing to blistering and occasional hospitalisation. The symptoms occur on exposed sites, can occur on cloudy days and sun exposure can cause severe reactions. It is more common in cystic fibrosis patients because they have frequent courses of drugs given at higher doses. Pseudoporphyria can arise with the fluoroquinolones.

The potential for fluoroquinolone-induced phototoxicity was highlighted in 1993, by the high incidence of reported photosensitivity reactions in patients treated with lomefloxacin. In clinical trials, there was a 2.5%–10% incidence of photosensitivity. The U.S. Adverse Drug Reaction Monitoring System showed 182 reports of photosensitivity for lomefloxacin from 25×10^3 prescriptions. The incidence for norfloxacin and ciprofloxacin was 19 from 10×10^6 and 29 from 31×10^6 prescriptions, respectively. Furthermore, photocarcinogenesis was reported in mice treated with lomefloxacin.

Results and Discussion

Although photochemistry is an inexact science, there are structure activity relationships that provide reasons to believe moxifloxacin is more photostable than lomefloxacin. Therefore, a study was designed to evaluate the photosensitising ability of moxifloxacin compared to lomefloxacin. The study was a prospective, intra-patient comparison of the effects of each medication compared to placebo. The treatments were administered in a randomised double blind manner.

The phototesting procedure used a monochrometer to expose specific sites on the patient's back to defined bands (30 nm) of wavelengths across the solar UVA spectrum and the visible blue region. The amount of exposure (mj/cm) to the defined waveband that elicited erythema was the chosen end point, and was defined as the minimal erythema dose (MED). Initially each patient was tested to determine that they were a normal reactor and the baseline MED was determined before treatment. Patients then received a seven-day treatment with one of the medications. Phototesting was repeated between day 5-day 7, at the time of stable pharmacokinetics, and at 2 day intervals after cessation of treatment. The objective was to see how the MED changed with the treatment.

The result from one study patient is displayed in Fig. 1, showing his reaction to lower doses in the UVA spectrum following treatment with 400 mg/day of lomefloxacin. A comparison of the MED for lomefloxacin, moxifloxacin and placebo at one specific wavelength (365 + 30 nm) is shown in Fig. 2. The decrease in MED after treatment with lomefloxacin was significant whereas treatment with either 200 mg/day, 400 mg/day of moxifloxacin or placebo produced no significant change. The photosensitivity was not long lasting; within 2 days of lomefloxacin withdrawal, the MED value was not significantly different from baseline.

Fig. 1
Illustration of response of one patient to treatment with 400 mg/kg of lomefloxacin followed by exposure to UVA irradiation

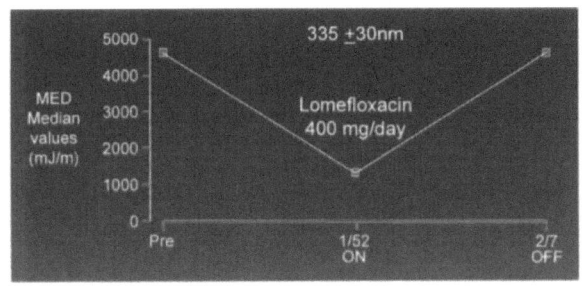

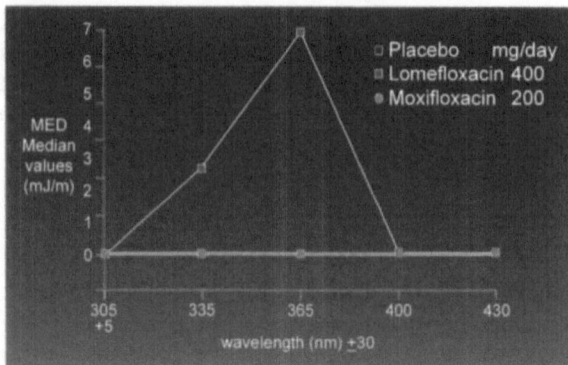

Fig. 2
The change in minimal erythema dose (MED) of patients treated with either lomefloxacin (400 mg/day) or moxifloxacin (200 mg/day or 400 mg/day) and then exposed to UVA irradiation (365 ± 30 nm)

Another way to express the data is the phototoxic index (P. I.) which is defined as at 365 + 30 mm as:

$$\text{Phototoxic index (P.I.)} = \frac{\text{baseline MED}}{\text{on therapy MED}}$$

The P. I. defines the degree of photosensitization due to a particular drug. The phototoxic indices for moxifloxacin and lomefloxacin across the UVA spectrum are shown in Fig. 3. The data show that lomefloxacin is phototoxic at wavelengths between 335 and 365 nm. By comparison, the P. I. of moxifloxacin was identical to placebo, indicating it did not cause photosensitivity. The P. I. can be used to categorise drugs as mild, moderate or severe inducers of phototoxicity. Among the fluoroquinolones, ciprofloxacin is mild with a P. I. of 1.4-3; lomefloxacin and sparfloxacin are moderate with a P. I. between 3-6; an earlier fluoroquinolone (BAY y 3118) had a P. I. about 30.

The P. I. is useful to illustrate the relative amount of time one can stay outdoors before erythema is induced by irradiation from sunlight. The amount of irradiation at 365 + 30 nm from sunlight was measured at mid-day in July in Dundee (56° N) and in Athens (40° N). From this data it was possible to predict the length of exposure to sunlight required to cause erythema in untreated patients and in those created with fluoroquinolones. Erythema would be in-

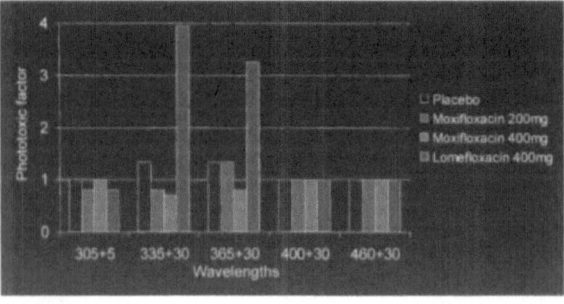

Fig. 3
The variation in phototoxic factor with wavelength of UVA irradiation in patients treated with either lomefloxacin (400 mg/day) or moxifloxacin (200 mg/day or 400 mg/day) and then exposed to irradiation 5–7 days post treatment

duced in 74 min in Dundee and 55 min in Athens for untreated patients. The time would be identical for patients on moxifloxacin due to its lack of phototoxicity. However, when treated with lomefloxacin, the exposure time to induce a reaction would be reduced to 12 min in Dundee and 9 min in Athens. Treated with a drug with a P.I. of 30 would decrease the required exposure to 2 min and 1 min, respectively. This indicates the significance of photosensitivity for patients treated with fluoroquinolones.

Conclusion

Phototoxicity among fluoroquinolones varies in severity, with minor changes in molecular structure. Lomefloxacin phototoxicity is characteristic of the fluoro-quinolones, is UVA dependent, is maximal at 24 h and clears within 48 h of stopping the drug. Phototoxicity produces erythema and can progress to blistering. Moxifloxacin did not demonstrate phototoxicity at 200 mg/day and 400 mg/day.

CHAPTER 26

Fluoroquinolone Safety and Tolerability   26

PETER BALL

Abstract. Fluoroquinolones in general have an excellent safety record. Adverse drug reactions primarily affect the gastrointestinal system, skin and CNS, occur at a frequency of around 5% or less and are almost invariably mild in severity. Most are considered class effects. Severe reactions, e.g. phototoxicity, renal syndromes and tendinitis, are rare. Certain fluoroquinolones (FQ) may cause structure-related effects associated with particular side chains, e.g. 8-halo-genation and severe phototoxicity, whilst others may produce idiosyncratic reactions which appear to be agent specific. The latter would include the haemolytic-uraemic syndrome associated with temafloxacin and, more recently, the severe and probably immunologically-mediated hepatic reactions observed with trovafloxacin. FQ developed in the 1990s have conformed to the usual class related effects, although certain agents, e.g. grepafloxacin (GI effects), trovafloxacin (CNS) and the 8-chloro derivatives, clinafloxacin and sitafloxacin (phototoxicity), have higher specific incidences. New phenomena, probably previously unrecognised as class effects, e.g. QTc prolongation and potential for pre-arrhythmic cardiac conduction anomalies, continue to appear. Moxifloxacin has been investigated in almost 5000 patients and, in this population, has been shown to have a low frequency of class-related ADRs and no novel phenomena.

Introduction

Over 15 years of clinical use, the fluoroquinolones have proved to be highly effective therapeutic agents with an excellent record of safety. The range of ADRs associated with FQ therapy have largely been reported with other antibiotic classes and include, gastrointestinal (GI) effects (nausea, diarrhoea and, rarely, pseudomembranous colitis), hypersensitivity reactions (maculo-papular rashes, urticaria and anaphylaxis), renal syndromes (nephritis and crystalluria), hepatic effects (cholestasis, hepatitis and hepatic failure) and CNS ADRs including, rarely, convulsions and psychoses. Comparative trials show the majority of FQ to have a similar safety record to beta-lactams and macrolides.

However, potentially serious effects, both idiosyncratic and class-related have infrequently occurred. These are summarised in Table 1. Although many of these effects were predicted from past experience of, and animal data on precursor compounds including nalidixic acid and its naphthyridine congeners, and early non-fluorinated quinolones, such as pipemidic and piromidic acids, some effects associated with the second and third generation fluoroquinolones could not have been anticipated. These include severe phototoxicity, tendinitis, the "temafloxacin syndrome", clinically significant QTc prolongation and severe hepatic syndromes.

Table 1. The potentially serious adverse drug reactions observed with fluoroquinolones

Effects	Agents implicated
Crystalluria	all (animals), tosufloxacin
Joint cartilage erosions	all (juvenile animals)
Severe tendinitis/rupture	all (pefloxacin, levofloxacin)
Phototoxicity	8-chloro derivatives
Photocarcinogenicity	lomefloxacin
Haemolytic-uraemic syndrome	temafloxacin
CNS disorders	ofloxacin, trovafloxacin
Cardiac conduction	sparfloxacin, grepafloxacin
Hepatic syndromes	all (trovafloxacin) (see text)

Incidence of common class effects

Investigation of the second generation fluoroquinolones, e. g. ciprofloxacin, nor-floxacin and ofloxacin, demonstrated overall ADR rates of 5–10%, evenly distributed between GI, skin and CNS phenomena at rates of 1–5%. Reports of later second generation and early third generation agents, commencing with fleroxacin and temafloxacin, show considerably higher incidences. However, these are largely explained by the innovative use of direct questioning and encouragement of patient reporting by questionnaires and other means. Thus, FQ developed in the 1990s are all associated with ADR rates of 25–50%. The relation of these effects to treatment is often poorly defined and considerably less than half of all ADRs are "probably" or "possibly" related. About a third of patients receiving moxifloxacin reported possible ADRs but the incidence of related effects was considerably less. ADR-associated – as opposed to treatment failure related – discontinuation rates may be a more sensitive measure of the true incidence of ADRs and are certainly a more rational basis for comparison between modern agents. Discontinuation rates for these agents are usually 2–4% but may be higher due to certain specific effects, e. g. dizziness (trovafloxacin) and taste per-version/nausea (grepafloxacin). The discontinuation rate for moxifloxacin was 3.8% and none of the class effects seen more commonly with contemporary agents, e.g. nausea, dizziness and rash, caused discontinuation in more than 1% of patients.

The major moxifloxacin-associated ADRs in clinical trials were nausea (7–8%), diarrhoea (5.7%), dizziness (2.9%) and headache (2%). Abdominal discomfort and dyspepsia were infrequent. With the exception of the higher rate of nausea, these incidences were similar to or less than those of comparators, and were independent of sex, age, race or syndrome treated.

More serious events reported during treatment with moxifloxacin included chest pain, dyspnoea, "pneumonia" and ventricular arrhythmias (none directly related to therapy). All occurred at similar frequency to comparators.

Specific fluoroquinolone adverse effects

Effects on the QT interval

Animal studies have shown that many FQ prolong the rate corrected electro-cardiographic QT interval (QTc). Rapid high dose infusion may precipitate pre-arrhythmic effects, e. g. Torsade de Pointes, and ventricular arrhythmias. Both sparfloxacin and grepafloxacin are reported to cause QTc prolongation in man and sparfloxacin therapy has been associated with ventricular arrhythmias, although their relation to therapy is questionable. Moxifloxacin may prolong the QTc interval, on average 4 msec, equal to the rates associated with comparator agents. QTc prolongation to > 500 msec (upper limit of normal 450–470 msec) was observed in 0.5 % of patients but no risk factors for arrhythmias (reverse rate depolarisation, Torsade de Pointes) or arrhythmias themselves were seen. Nevertheless, caution will be required in patients receiving other agents known to prolong the QTc intervals, e. g. class I/III anti-arrhythmics or terfenadine.

For other newer FQ there are less data. There are no available animal studies or published human data on trovafloxacin, levofloxacin or gatifloxacin. CPMP data in Europe suggest that there were no cases of QTc prolongation of > 50 msec or to > 450 msec with trovafloxacin. No arrhythmias have been reported with either trovafloxacin or levofloxacin, although a small number of cases of Torsade de Pointes associated with the latter were reported to the FDA Adverse Event Reporting System.

CNS events

In the past, higher levels of CNS ADRs were reported with lomefloxacin (convulsions), norfloxacin (dizziness) and ofloxacin (sleep disturbance, confusion and psychological effects). For sparfloxacin and grepafloxacin, frequencies of 5–6 % are reported compared with 3 % for moxifloxacin. In clinical trials, trovafloxacin had an incidence of dizziness of up to 11 % (mostly as a first dose light headedness effect in young women) although the overall incidence of CNS effects was around 7 %. Dizziness has been reported in 2.9 % of patients receiving moxifloxacin. Post marketing surveillance data from the USA has shown a higher incidence of other trovafloxacin associated CNS effects, e. g. confusion and sleep disturbance, compared with levofloxacin and other FQ.

Differential GABA and NMDA receptor binding affinities may explain the differences in CNS ADR rates and the potential for interaction with other CNS reacting agents such as theophylline and the NSAIDs.

Hepatic reactions

Various reactions, ranging in severity from transaminase elevations, through hepatitis, to liver failure, have been reported with fluoroquinolones. Mild transaminase elevations to 1.5–3 times upper limit of normal are observed in 1–5% of patients (moxifloxacin 3%). Serious hepatic ADRs are rare.

However, post-marketing surveillance has indicated a higher frequency of unpredictable hepatic events with trovafloxacin. Clinically significant, severe reactions, including a small number of related deaths and transplants, have occurred. A third of patients with hepatic reactions have shown evidence of hypersensitivity, a similar proportion had a pre-exisiting liver or biliary disorder which might have predisposed to the event and half were receiving concomitant therapy which possibly contributed to hepatototxicity. Eosinophilic hepatitis has been observed on liver biopsy.

The incidence of severe hepatic reactions to trovafloxacin is approximately 0.005%. This is not very significantly different from that of penicillin anaphylaxis or chloramphenicol-induced aplasia (0.002–0.005%), or of the cholestatic hepatitis syndromes induced by co-amoxiclav or flucloxacillin. Nevertheless, The European Registration Authority (CPMP) ordered the suspension of the trovafloxacin license in June 1999. In the USA the FDA have recommended restriction to life or limb-threatening infections, treated in hospital, initially intravenously, in patients for whom no alternatives exist.

Phototoxicity

Severe phototoxicity is associated with halogenation at the 8 position of the fluoroquinolone nucleus. This has proved a particular problem with 8-chloro derivatives and has resulted in the discontinuation (Bay y 3118) or retardation (clinafloxacin, sitafloxacin) of some very potent new agents. Newer compounds with similarly potent activity but alternate 8-substitutions, e.g. moxifloxacin, trovafloxacin and gemifloxacin produce only mild phototoxic reactions in <0.05%.

Other reactions

Tendinitis, possibly still most commonly reported with pefloxacin, is a rare event associated with all of the currently available fluoroquinolones. It is more common in the elderly and in those receiving corticosteroid therapy. Anaphylactic reactions are also a class effect, more common in AIDS or CF patients. More recently, trovafloxacin-associated pancreatitis has been reported.

Conclusions

Recent events have questioned knowledge of the structure-ADR relationships of the quinolone group. In particular, there is speculation that either the 1-difluorophenyl side chain unique to temafloxacin and trovafloxacin, or the possession of a naphthyridine (as opposed to fluoroquinolone) nucleus, may prove more reactogenic than other configurations. There is little evidence for either hypothesis. For example, neither enoxacin nor tosufloxacin, both naphthyridines, appear to have been associated with an abnormal incidence of hepatic reactions.

However, it is certain that registration authorities will now look even more closely at the data on fluoroquinolones and naphthyridones currently in development. Class labeling may alter to reflect QTc effects and possible major organ toxicity.

The renaissance of the fluoroquinolone group in the 1990s, led by compounds with increasingly more potent activity against the pneumococcus, has thus received a number of challenges. These have largely related to specific compounds and have led to their restriction/suspension (e.g. trovafloxacin) or withdrawal (e.g. Bay y 3118, temafloxacin). The remaining agents retain the safety features more characteristic of the group as a whole. Of those agents which are now or will be available by the millennium, levofloxacin suffers from lesser activity and a complex dosing schedule relating to predominant renal excretion, sparfloxacin has essentially been abandoned due to phototoxicity and possible QTc related arrhythmias, grepafloxacin is poorly tolerated due to taste perversion and nausea and clinafloxacin has serious phototoxicity problems. Of the existing second generation agents, ciprofloxacin has an impressive safety record but suffers from perceptions of inactivity against the pneumococcus. Trovafloxacin, which has significantly improved anti-Gram-positive activity, appeared the ideal agent to supplement existing FQ agents in the respiratory tract, but has been compromised by rare but severe hepatotoxicity. Moxifloxacin is now ideally placed to assume this role, having equivalent potency, better PK/PD and excellent clinical efficacy with no evidence of serious toxicity. There is little data available on other compounds in development, but the year 2000 looks to be yet another interesting waypoint in the saga of the fluoroquinolone group.

References

Ball P (1998) The quinolones: history and overview. In: The Quinolones, VT Andriole (Ed), Academic Press, pp 1–28

Ball P, Tillotson GS (1995) Tolerability of fluoroquinolone antibiotics: past, present and future. Drug Safety 13:343–358

Ball P, Fernald A, Tillotson GS (1998) Therapeutic advances of new fluoroquinolones. Exp Opin Invest Drugs 7:761–783

Ball, P, Mandell L, Niki Y, Tillotson G (1999) Comparative tolerability of the newer fluoroquinolone antibacterials. Drug Safety (in press)

Blum MD, Graham DJ, McCloskey CA (1994) Temafloxacin syndrome: review of 95 cases. Clin Infect Dis 18:946–950

Davis R, Bryson HM (1994) Levofloxacin: a review of its antibacterial activity, pharmacokinetics and therapeutic efficacy. Drugs 47:677–700

Domagala JM (1994) Structure-activity and structure-side-effect relationships for the fluoroquinolone antibacterials. J Antimicrob Chemother 33:685–706

Hayem G et al. (1995) A reappraisal of quinolone tolerability. The experience of their musculoskeletal adverse effects. Drug Saf 13:338–342

Lipsky BA, Baker CA (1999) Fluoroquinolone toxicity profiles: a review focusing on newer agents. Clin Infect Dis 28:352–364

Rizk E (1992) The US clinical experience with lomefloxacin, a new once daily fluoroquinolone. Am J Med (Suppl 4A):130S–1305S

Rubinstein E (1996) Safety profile of sparfloxacin in the treatment of respiratory tract infections. J Antimicrob Chemother 37 (Suppl A):145–160

Stahlmann R, Schwabe R (1997) Safety profile of grepafloxacin compared with other fluoroquinolones. J Antimicrob Chemother 40 (Suppl A):83–92

Williams D, Hopkins S (1998) Safety of trovafloxacin in treatment of lower respiratory tract infections. Eur J Clin Microbiol Infect Dis 17:454–458

Part 4
Clinical Needs in the Millenium

CHAPTER 27

Clinical Needs in the Millennium – Community Acquired Pneumonia

PAUL LÉOPHONTE

Abstract. Community-acquired pneumonia (CAP) is a major global public health problem. The incidence is 1 – 11.6/1000 in the general population; mortality is 0.5 – 1.4 million/year (WHO). The main pathogens are *Streptococcus pneumoniae, Haemophilus influenzae, Mycoplasma pneumoniae, Chlamydia sp., Legionella pneumophila* and viruses. The prevalence of antibiotic-resistant *S. pneumoniae* and *H. influenzae* is increasing dramatically worldwide. Scoring systems to predict risk of mortality have been proposed to determine when to refer a patient to hospital. Guidelines for empiric antibiotic treatment have been developed in many countries. Beta-lactams and/or macrolides are generally recommended, but they have limitations, including inadequate spectrum of activity and emerging development of resistance.

In the new millennium, we need to better our knowledge regarding causative pathogens of outpatient pneumonia and undetermined cases; to reduce antibiotic resistance rates and the spread of resistant strains; to develop an easy-to-use scoring system, especially for moderate pneumonia; and we need to determine precise indications for new fluoroquinolones which are effective against the main causative pathogens of CAP.

Introduction

Community acquired pneumonia (CAP), as distinguished from that acquired nosocomially or in a long term facility, is an acute infection of the lung parenchyma accompanied by altered breath sounds and/or rales and associated with some symptoms of acute lower respiratory tract infection such as fever or hypothermia, rigors, sweats, new cough with or without sputum production or change in the colour of respiratory secretions in a patient with a chronic cough, chest discomfort, or the onset of dyspnea and nonspecific symptoms such as fatigue, myalgias, abdominal pain, anorexia and headache [1].

The incidence of CAP has been evaluated in the general population as being between 1 and 11.6/1000 annually, increasing with age (at 65 years, 25 to 44/1000 annually) and co-morbidities [2]. Four million cases occur annually in the USA and 1 to 3 million cases in Europe (UK, France, Italy, Germany and Spain). The mean percentage of patients hospitalised is between 17 and 35%. Overall mortality is estimated at between 1 and 3%: <1% in patients who are not hospitalised, increasing to 6–24% among hospitalised patients, and 22–57% in intensive care units [3]. In the USA, during the first part of this century, there was a dramatic decrease in mortality from 180 deaths/100,000 (1900) to 20/100,000 (1950) which remained relatively stable until 1979 when the death rate started to increase [4]. This was attributed mainly to the greater proportion of persons over 65 years of age, but as age adjusted rates also increased, other factors, such as the proportion of the population with underlying medical conditions (active malignancies, immunosuppression, neurological disease, congestive heart failure, diabetes mellitus, AIDS), were thought to be contributing to the changing epidemiology. Mortality has been evaluated worldwide by the WHO to be between 500,000 and 1.4 million deaths per year.

Prospective studies of CAP in hospitalised patients have failed to identify a causative agent in 40–60% of cases. The most common etiological agent was *Streptococcus pneumoniae*, accounting for approximately two-thirds of the cases of pneumonia [5]. *Chlamydia pneumoniae* was implicated as a second major cause of CAP in some studies [6]. Other pathogens implicated less frequently include *Mycoplasma pneumoniae, Legionella pneumophila, Coxiella burnetii* and viruses. The incidence of *L. pneumophila, Haemophilus influenzae*, Gram-negative enterobacteria, *Moraxella catarrhalis* and *Staphylococcus aureus* increase in the elderly and patients with co-morbidities. Similar pathogens have been recorded in smaller outpatient studies, but with a greater incidence of *M. pneumoniae* and *C. pneumoniae*, particularly amongst younger patients (Fig. 1).

In suspected CAP, antimicrobial therapy is indicated and a chest radiograph demonstrating the presence of an acute infiltrate will establish diagnosis. It has been suggested that a chest X-ray is of value in only a minority of community based patients with LRTI, in patients with focal chest signs or after failure of first line therapy [5].

No convincing association has been demonstrated between individual symptoms, physical findings of laboratory test results and specific aetiology in the evaluation of CAP although acute onset, single shaking chill (rigor) and alveolar consolidation are common features of pneumococcal pneumonia. In one study a combination of variables including cardiovascular disease, acute onset of illness, pleuritic pain, Gram-positive bacteria in sputum, and leukocyte count distinguished correctly between pneumococci and others in 80% of cases [7].

The prognosis of patients with CAP ranges from rapid recovery to death, which can occur early in the course of the disease. The assessment of severity of disease is important in guiding decisions regarding hospital admission, admission to ICU and antibiotic treatment. The great variability seen in rates of hospital admission and lengths of stay for pneumonia in part reflects uncertainty among physicians in assessing the severity of the illness and the perceived benefits of hospital care.

Various scoring systems have been proposed to predict the risk of mortality and to identify patients at low risk for morbidity or mortality. The most recent system is a prediction rule to identify patients with CAP who are at risk of death and other adverse outcomes by examining demographic and clinical factors [8]. Patients are stratified into 5 classes using a cumulative point system based on 19 variables, including age, gender, nursing home residence, co-morbid illness, signs and symptoms and laboratory test abnormalities. Category 1 and 2 patients have a low risk of mortality (<1%) and can be treated as outpatients with oral antimicrobial agents; category 3 patients, with a higher mortality rate, should be observed for 24–48 hours in hospital before being allowed home as outpatients;

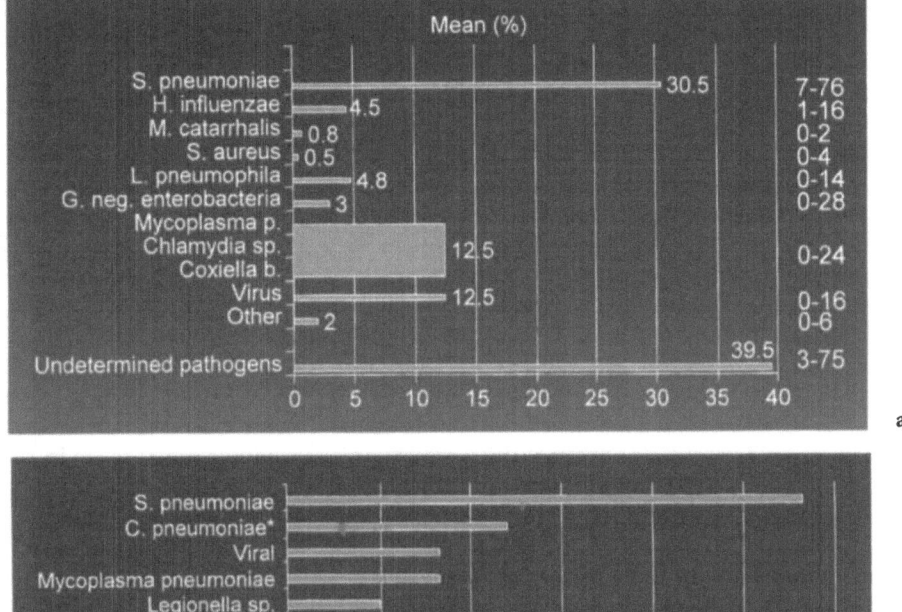

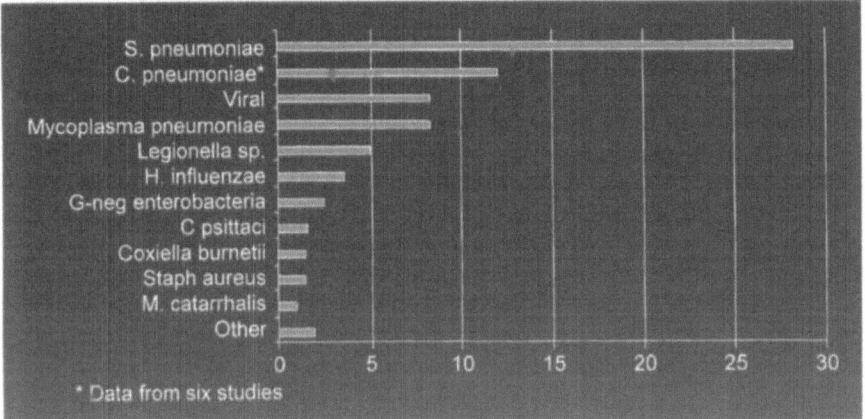

Fig. 1 The epidemiology of community acquired pneumonia. Data (**a**) from 21 studies (4982 patients) and data (**b**) from 26 studies (5961 patients)

category 4 and 5 patients (mortality rates, 10% and 30%, respectively) should be hospitalised to receive parenteral treatment. The rule has not been evaluated prospectively by general practitioners, among outpatients and is limited by over-simplification. Patients designated as low risk may have important medical and psychosocial contraindications to outpatient care such as inadequate social support, low compliance, drug abuse; patients with rare conditions (neuromuscular disease, immunosuppression) are not included as predictors but have an increased risk of a poor outcome. A scoring system for moderate cases, between benign pneumonia and severely ill patients that is easy to use in routine clinical practice is necessary.

Strategies that reduce the use of traditional hospital care may result in huge cost savings and a reduction in the rate of hospitalisation of low risk patients is consistent with clear preferences to be treated at home.

Initial antimicrobial therapy is generally empirical. The selection of an anti-microbial agent in the absence of an etiological agent is based on multiple variables including severity of illness, patient age, antimicrobial intolerance or side effects, clinical features, co-morbidities, concomitant medications, exposure and epidemiological setting. Inadequate antibiotic therapy is a factor of poor prognosis [9].

Guidelines for the empiric treatment of CAP vary in different countries. They include the use of penicillins, macrolides and aminopenicillins in patients without risk factors; broad spectrum antibiotics like cephalosporins, sometimes in association with macrolides or Co-amoxyclavulanic acid, in patients with risk factors [10, 11]. However, a survey of initial antibiotic therapy of CAP in 5 European countries among general practitioners has demonstrated that these guidelines are not always adhered to. Large differences in antimicrobial usage exist [12]: high usage of aminopenicillins in France (38%) and UK (35%); penicillins (11%) and tetracyclines (9%) in Germany; macrolides (41%) in Spain; and cephalosporins (54%) and third generation cephalosporins (45%) in Italy (Table 1).

Resistance to antibiotics commonly prescribed for CAP is increasing at an alarming rate. The Alexander Project 1992–1996 confirmed that the clinical utility of penicillin, macrolides and other classes of antimicrobials is seriously compromised by the increasing prevalence of resistance to these compounds among clinical isolates of *S. pneumoniae* in many countries worldwide [13]. The high rates of penicillin resistance found in Spain in the early 1990s are now apparent in France, USA and China, and there is evidence of evolution of resistance in other countries around the world (Table 2). Penicillin resistance in pneumococci occurs as a result of alterations in the high molecular weight penicillin binding proteins (PBP). Since these are also targets for aminopenicillins, cepha-

Table 1. The antibiotics used for initial therapy of community-acquired pneumonia in European countries

	Initial Therapy (%)				
	France	UK	Germany	Spain	Italy
Aminopenicillin	37.7	35	15.8	14.7	10.8
Coamoxiclav	19.7	14	3.4	8.8	3.1
Cephalosporins	24.5	17.4	10	16.2	53.8
Third-generation cephalosporins	16.4	0	2.2	0	44.6
Penicillin	0	1.2	11.2	0	3.1
Macrolides	21.3	23.3	28.1	41.2	12.3
Tetracyclines	1.6	0	9	0	0
Fluoroquinolones	4.9	11.7	11.2	14.7	4.6
SMX-TMP	0	3.5	1.1	0	0

Table 2. The increasing global prevalence of penicillin-resistant *Streptococcus pneumoniae*

		MIC (0.12–1 mg/L)	MIC (≥2 mg/L)
UK	(London)	6	6
France	(Toulouse)	20	29
Spain	(Barcelona)	17	35
Germany	(Weingarten)	15	0
Italy	(Genova)	4	3
USA	(New York)	13	27
South Africa	(Johannesburg)	26	5
China	(Hong Kong)	5	56

Table 3
The increasing global prevalence of macrolide-resistant *Streptococcus pneumoniae*

		MIC (>1 mg/L)
UK	(London)	7
France	(Toulouse)	46
Spain	(Barcelona)	33
Germany	(Weingarten)	6
Italy	(Genova)	30
USA	(New York)	16
South Africa	(Johannesburg)	8
China	(Hong Kong)	78

losporins and carbapenems, the activity of these compounds is also diminished against pneumococci which are not fully susceptible to penicillin. Macrolide resistance, particularly in France, Spain, Italy and China, is increasing both in association with and independently of penicillin resistance (Table 3).

The production of beta-lactamase to *H. influenzae* is widespread but varies considerably (Table 4): China (38%); USA, Spain, France and Belgium (20–30%); UK and Czech Republic (14.2%, 13%); Netherlands, Germany (<10%).

The main antimicrobial agents used in the treatment of CAP are beta-lactams and/or macrolides. They are effective and safe but have a limited spectrum of activity against the main causative pathogens. Beta-lactams are not active against *L. pneumophila* and *M. pneumoniae* and, with increased resistance, are not always active against *S. pneumoniae* and *H. influenzae*. Macrolides are effective against the atypical pathogens, *L. pneumophila*, *C. pneumoniae* and *M. pneumoniae*, but are inactive against *H. influenzae*, and a high percentage of *S. pneumoniae* are resistant. In controlled, randomised clinical trials the newer macrolides (azithromycin, clarithromycin) and newer fluoroquinolones (levo-

Table 4. The prevalence of antibiotic-resistant *Haemophilus influenzae*

		β-lactam+	Cefaclor	Chloramph.	Cotrimox.
UK	(London)	9	3.4	0.7	7.3
France	(Toulouse)	19.5	4.1	0	0.4
Spain	(Barcelona)	30	11.1	4.4	12.2
Germany	(Weingarten)	3.5	3	0	0.4
Italy	(Genova)	5.4	1.7	1.4	1.1
USA	(New York)	19.7	1.9	0	0

Chloramp. – chloramphenical, Cotrimox – cotrimoxazole

Table 5. Spectrum of various antibotic treatments of community acquired pneumonia

	L. pneumophila	*M. pneumoniae*	*S. pneumoniae*	*H. influenzae*
β-lactam	–	–	±	±
Macrolides	+	+	±	–
Fluoroquinolones	+	+	±	+
New Fluoroquinolones	+	+	+	+

floxacin, trovafloxacin, grepafloxacin) have been shown to be comparable to standard beta-lactam agents for empiric therapy of CAP. They have also been shown to be superior to erythromycin in vitro against the atypical pathogens, with fewer gastrointestinal side effects [14]. The fluoroquinolones show enhanced in vitro activity against *S. pneumoniae* (including penicillin resistant strains, *H. influenzae*, *Legionella* spp., *M. pneumoniae* and *C. pneumoniae*. The precise indications for new fluoroquinolones (efficacy, response time and rate, cure and return to work) need to be defined against all the main causative pathogens of CAP (Table 5).

Looking to the future, a greater knowledge of the causative organisms in outpatient pneumonia and pneumonias with specific co-morbidities and improved methods for determining aetiologies of unknown origin will enhance patient morbidity and mortality. There is a need to reduce the resistance rates and spread of respiratory pathogens associated with CAP through improved compliance programs, international control teams, more judicious use 'of antibiotics (non-medical use, inappropriate indications, prescribing guidelines) and implementation of preventative measures including vaccination programmes.

References

1. File TM Jr., Barttett JG, Breumann RG, Mandell LA (1998) Community acquired pneumonia in Adults: Guidelines for management. Clinical Infect Dis 26:811–838
2. Niederman MS, Fein AM (1986) Pneumonia in the elderly. Clin Geriatr Med 2(2):241–268
3. Marrie TJ (1994) Community acquired pneumonia. Clin Infect Dis 18(4):501–513
4. Gilbert K, Fine MJ (1994) Assessing prognosis and predicting patient outcomes in community acquired pneumonia Semin Respir Infect 9(3):140–152
5. Huchon G, Woodhead M (1998) Management of adult community-acquired lower respiratory tract infection. Eur Respir Rev 391–425
6. Woodhead MA (1998) Community-acquired pneumonia guidelines – an international comparison: a view from Europe. Chest 113(3):183S–187S
7. Bohte R, Hermans J, van de Broek PJ (1996) Early recognition of Streptococcus pneumoniae in patients with community acquired pneumonia. Eur J Clin Microbiol Infect Dis 15:201–205
8. Fine MJ, Auble TE, Yealy DM et al. (1997) A prediction rule to identify low-risk patients with community acquired pneumonia. NEJM 336(4):243–250
9. Torres A, Serra Balles J, Ferrer A et al. (1991) Severe community acquired pneumonia. Epidemiology and prognosis factors. Am Rev Respir Dis 144:311–318
10. Tremolieres F (1998) Lettre Infectiol. 13:220–228
11. American Thoracic Society 1993. Guidelines for the initial management of adults with community-acquired pneumonia: diagnosis, assessment of severity and initial antimicrobial therapy. Am Rev Respir Dis 148:1418–1426
12. Huchon GJ, Gialdroni-Grassi G, Leophonte P, Manresa F, Schaberg T, Woodhead M (1996) Initial antibiotic therapy for lower respiratory tract infection in the community: a European survey. Eur Resp 9(8):1590–1595
13. Felmingham D, Washington J, The Alexander Project Group (1999) Trends in the antimicrobial susceptibilitiy of bacterial respiratory tract pathogens – Findings of the Alexander Project 1992–1996. J Chemother 11(1):5–22
14. Yu VL, Vergis, EN (1998) New macrolides or new quinolones as monotherapy for patients with community-acquired pnuemonia. Our cup runneth over? Chest 113:1158–1159

CHAPTER 28

Clinical Needs in The Millennium – Pneumonia – The Role of Moxifloxacin

MARTIN SPRINGSKLEE

Abstract. Four clinical studies were conducted in over 30 countries with patients suffering from community-acquired pneumonia. Moxifloxacin (400 mg qd 10 d) was compared to clarithromycin (500 mg bid 10 d) or amoxicillin (1 g tid 10 d) all treatment was oral. Clinical results at first visit post therapy demonstrated 94.4 % success among patients treated with moxifloxacin, compared with 92.9 % among those who received clarithromycin or amoxicillin. Bacteriological response in the moxifloxacin group achieved 91 %, which included 94 % eradication of penicillin-resistant *S. pneumoniae* (MIC ≥ 1.0) (17/18 patients) and complete eradication of clarithromycin-resistant *S. pneumoniae* (MIC ≥ 8.0) (26/26 patients).

Introduction

Streptococcus pneumoniae is one of the most common aetiological agents associated with community acquired pneumonia (CAP). Moxifloxacin is highly active against clinical isolates of *S. pneumoniae* [1] collected worldwide (MIC: 0.06–0.12; MIC_{90}: 0.12 µg/mL). Activity was found to be independent of the source of the isolates. Strains from hospitalised patients were as susceptible as strains from outpatients; MIC values were independent of the geographic origin of the strains; those from the main foci of penicillin resistance were not different in their susceptibilities to moxifloxacin than those from countries with a low prevalence of penicillin resistance.

Moxifloxacin is more active in vitro against *S. pneumoniae* than most other fluoroquinolones, irrespective of the level of penicillin and macrolide resistance. It exhibits the highest antibacterial activity in terms of MIC_{90} (<0.12 µg/mL), half that of sparfloxacin and 4-8 fold more active than ciprofloxacin, ofloxacin and levofloxacin [2]. In-vitro pharmacodynamic models have shown moxifloxacin to be rapidly bactericidal against strains of *S. pneumoniae*, with rates of bacterial killing exceeding those of levofloxacin and sparfloxacin [3].

Moxifloxacin is highly active in vitro against *Haemophilus influenzae* (MIC_{90} 0.12 µg/mL) and susceptibility is independent from beta-lactamase production. Simulation of human serum kinetics (400 mg po) in a pharmacodynamic model have demonstrated that *H. influenzae* was eliminated within 8 h and laboratory generated isogenic mutants, with increased MIC values, were killed less rapidly, but were eliminated within 24 h [4].

Moxifloxacin shows excellent in-vitro activity against *Moraxella catarrhalis* (0.12 µg/mL) and *Staphylococcus aureus* (0.12 µg/mL) and atypical pathogens,

Mycoplasma pneumoniae (MIC_{90} 0.06 µg/mL), *Chlamydia pneumoniae* (0.06 µg/mL) and *Legionella pneumophila* [5, 6].

Data from animal and human studies show that moxifloxacin achieves extensive penetration into lung tissue: the concentration of moxifloxacin exceeds the MIC_{90} of the common respiratory pathogens in alveolar macrophages, bronchial mucosa and epithelial lining fluid [7].

Clinical trials were undertaken to corroborate the excellent preclinical/pharmacokinetic profile of moxifloxacin as an important new antibiotic in the treatment of CAP.

Results and Discussion

The role of moxifloxacin in the treatment of CAP has been investigated in five clinical studies (3 randomised, double blind, comparative, phase III trials, one randomised, double blind, Phase II trial and one open non-comparative trial). These were all regulatory trials performed according to FDA, IDSA and EMEA guidelines and involved 1817 patients, 1144 of whom were treated with moxifloxacin.

Enrolment criteria included fever and or leucocytosis and or left shift, a positive chest X-ray with a new infiltrate, and one or more of the following: productive cough, purulent sputum, dyspnea or tachypnea, rigors or chills, pleuritic pain and rales or rhonchii indicating pneumonic consolidation.

The primary efficacy variable was clinical response at 3 – 5 days after the end of therapy. In some cases, a secondary variable was clinical response 2 – 4 days and 21 – 28 days after the end of therapy. Initial bacteriological identification of the pathogens isolated from patients was confirmed by a central laboratory. Atypical pathogens were identified by serology alone in two studies and by serology and culture in another two studies.

Study 119 was a phase III study to compare 200 mg and 400 mg moxifloxacin once daily with 500 mg clarithromycin twice daily for 10 days in 675 patients in South Africa, Europe and Southeast Asia. Study 130 was a phase III comparison of 400 mg moxifloxacin once daily with 500 mg clarithromycin twice daily for 10 days in 473 patients in USA. Study 129 was a non-comparative study of 400 mg moxifloxacin once daily for 10 days in 254 patients in USA. Study 140 was a phase II study to compare 400 mg moxifloxacin once daily with 1 g amoxicillin three times daily for 10 days in 408 patients in South Africa, Europe and USA. The clinical response data are presented in Table 1.

In study 119, the clinical response of 200 mg moxifloxacin once daily for 5 to 14 days was 94 % while that of 400 mg moxifloxacin was 94 % and the comparator, 500 mg amoxicillin three times daily (94 %). In study 130, the clinical response of 400 mg moxifloxacin once daily for 10 days (95 %) was also identical to the comparator, 500 mg clarithromycin twice daily (95 %). In a similar study, 140, the clinical response to moxifloxacin (92 %) was slightly higher than 1 g amoxicillin three times daily for 10 days (90 %). Clinical response to 400 mg moxifloxacin once daily for 10 days in the non-comparative trial was 97 %. Overall, the clinical response rate of 400 mg moxifloxacin was 94.4 % which was similar to the comparators 92.9 %.

Table 1. The clinical response in four trials of community acquired pneumonia shown comparing moxifloxacin against amoxicillin and clarithromycin

Study	200 mg	400 mg	Comparator	
119	169/180 (94)	167/177 (94)	164/174 (94)	Cla. 500 bid
130	–	173/183 (95)	173/182 (95)	Cla. 500 bid
129	–	184/190 (97)	–	
140	–	162/177 (92)	166/185 (90)	Amox. 1 g tid
Overall	(94)	686/727 (94.4)	503/541 (92.9)	

Cla. – clarithromycin, Amox. – amoxicillin

The secondary parameter, the combined clinical response rate at 2–4 days and 21–28 days after the end of therapy, was similar but slightly less than that of the clinical response at the first post therapy visit.

The clinical success rate of treatment with moxifloxacin in patients with positive serology for atypical pathogens (*M. pneumoniae, C. pneumoniae, L. pneumophila* and *Coxiella burnetti*) was similar to that of clarithromycin and was above 90 % in most cases (see Table 2).

The two major pathogens isolated were *S. pneumoniae* and *H. influenzae*. The bacteriological success rate (Table 3) at first post therapy visit in patients with isolates of *S. pneumoniae* 93/100 (93 %) with 400 mg moxifloxacin, higher than that of the comparators, 68/77 (88 %). Eradication rates were higher for moxifloxacin than for the comparators in patients with isolates of *H. influenzae*;

Table 2. The clinical response of patients who had positive serology for atypical pathogens after treatment with moxifloxacin

Success (%) in patients with positive serology for atypicals				
Pathogen	Moxi		Clari	Amox
	200 mg	400 mg	500 mg	1 g
M. pneumoniae	26/28 (93)	79/84 (94)	50/52 (96)	12/13 (92)
C. pneumoniae	13/15 (87)	126/136 (93)	69/72 (96)	1/1 (100)
L. pneumophila	–	4/4	3/4	1/2
C. burnetti	2/2	1/1	1/1	–

Table 3. The bacteriological success rates in patients treated with either moxifloxacin or comparative medications

Bacteriological success (%) – at first visit post-therapy		
	400 mg	Comparators
S. pneumoniae	93/100 (93)	68/77 (88)
H. influenzae	56/57 (98)	36/44 (82)

56/57 (98%) treated with 400 mg moxifloxacin; in comparison with the comparators, 36/44 (82%).

The bacteriological success rate in patients treated with 400 mg moxifloxacin, from whom a penicillin resistant S. pneumoniae (MIC ≥ 1.0) were isolated was 17/18 (94%) and a clarithromycin resistant S. pneumoniae (MIC ≥ 8.0) were 26/26 (100%).

Overall, 30% of the patients were microbiologically valid and 44% (126/289) of these bacteriological isolates were identified as S. pneumoniae. The MIC_{90} of moxifloxacin was 0.125 µg/mL, identical to the MIC values reported from in-vitro studies. Forty-two of 289 (15%) pathogens were isolated from blood and 32 (76%) of these isolates were S. pneumoniae. Thus 25% of all the S. pneumoniae isolates were cultured from blood. No positive blood culture was identified in any patient during or after treatment with moxifloxacin.

Two patients had a clinical outcome deemed as a non-success after receiving a full course of 10-day treatment. There was no indication of any progression to a septic or more severe course. In the comparator groups, a positive culture of Staphylococcus aureus was identified in one patient after initiation of clarithromycin therapy and a positive culture of Klebsiella pneumoniae was identified in one patient after initiation of amoxicillin therapy, not unexpected from a population of outpatients with moderately severe infections.

In conclusion, moxifloxacin exhibits excellent in-vitro activity against all the typical and atypical pathogens associated with CAP, particularly S. pneumoniae. The MIC_{90} of moxifloxacin was 0.125 µg/mL among the clinical S. pneumoniae isolates, identical to the MIC_{90} values reported from in-vitro studies. Clinical responses among drug susceptible and resistant S. pneumoniae indicate that the in-vitro profile of moxifloxacin is being translated into clinical practice. Treatment of patients with CAP with 400 mg moxifloxacin once daily for 10 days resulted in an overall clinical response of 94.4% and bacteriological response of 91%. It can be concluded from these initial data that moxifloxacin shows excellent clinical and bacteriological efficacy which is noticeably independent from resistance to beta-lactams or macrolides.

References

1. Dalhoff A (1998) Moxifloxacin- Review of microbiology. Antipneumococcal activity. In: Programme and Abstracts of the 6th International Symposium on New Quinolones, Denver, p 56
2. Marchese A, Debbia EA, Schito GC (1998) Comparative activity of Bay 12-8039 and other fluoroquinolones on clinical Streptococcus pneumoniae strains. Poster at ECC Hamburg
3. Lister PD, Sanders CC (1998) Pharmacodynamics of moxifloxacin against Streptococcus pneumoniae in an in vitro pharmacokinetic model. Poster at ICAAC San Diego, Abstract No. A21
4. Dalhoff A (1998) Moxifloxacin-review of microbiology. Activity against H. influenzae and H. parainfluenzae. In: Programme and Abstracts of the 6th International Symposium on New Quinolones, Denver
5. Focht J (1998) In vitro activity of Bay 12-8039 compared with other fluoroquinolones against bacterial strains from upper and lower respiratory tract infections in general practice. Poster ICID Boston 1998
6. Wise R, Andrews JM, Brenwald N (1996) In vitro activity of a new 8-methoxyquinolone Bay 12-8039 in comparison with other fluoroquinolones and B-lactams against recent isolates of Chlamydia. Poster at ICAAC New Orleans
7. Andrews J, Honeybourne D, Jevons G, Wise R (1998) Penetration of moxifloxacin into bronchial mucosa, epithelial lining fluid and alveolar macrophages following a single, 400 mg oral dose. Poster at IAAC San Diego, Abstract No. A29

Chapter 29

Clinical Needs in the Millenium – Acute Exacerbations of Chronic Bronchitis

Robert Wilson

Abstract. Acute exacerbations of chronic bronchitis (AECB) are common causes of community and hospital consultations, and have a major impact on patients' quality of life. The causes of AECB are multifactorial, including allergens, pollution, viral, and in $^1/_2$ to $^2/_3$ of cases, bacterial infections are involved. The major bacterial pathogens are *Haemophilus influenzae*, *Moraxella catarrhalis* and *Streptococcus pneumoniae*. Placebo-controlled trials show benefits from antibiotic treatment in patients with AECB and increased dyspnea, sputum volume and purulence. Some patients have bacterial colonisation of the lower respiratory tract during a stable state. The effect of this on bronchial inflammation and risk of further exacerbations has not been determined. Future antibiotic trials should seek to investigate whether increased potency *in vitro* translates into more rapid clinical response, improved quality of life or longer periods between acute exacerbations.

Introduction

Chronic obstructive pulmonary disease (COPD) represents a heterogeneous group of clinical conditions in which expiratory air flow obstruction is relatively fixed in comparison to asthma. Although patients may have a dominant pathology – chronic bronchitis, emphysema or airflow obstruction – all components may be present in different degrees.

Chronic bronchitis is defined as a chronic cough with sputum production on most days during at least 3 months per year over a period of two or more successive years. Those affected are subject to recurrent acute exacerbations characterised by symptoms of increased dyspnea, increased sputum volume and increased sputum purulence. Patients frequently develop generalised progressive small airways obstruction with relentless loss of ventilatory function, particularly if they continue to smoke cigarettes [1].

The cause of an acute exacerbation of chronic bronchitis (AECB) is multifactorial and includes allergens, air pollution, cigarette smoke and viral infections. Bacterial infection is present in about one-half to two thirds of cases. Causes may overlap: a primary viral upper respiratory infection with a secondary bacterial infection.

Results and Discussion

Differentiation of the cause of an AECB would lead to appropriate therapy, but in clinical practice it is often difficult to identify those patients in which significant bacterial infection is present. A study among general practitioners showed that most give attention to the sputum and its colour when making a decision[2]. Positive sputum culture by standard techniques only occurs in 50% of patients with AECB and sputum expectorated through the oropharynx may be contaminated with bacterial organisms such as *Haemophilus influenzae* and upper respiratory tract commensals found there.

In a recent study [3], 40 patients with stable COPD were subjected to a protected specimen brush (PSB) biopsy during bronchoscopy. Ten patients (25%), were shown to have chronic colonisation in the lower airways when the patients were well; a positive PSB (>1000 cfu/mL) with pathogens including *H. influenzae* (6), *Streptococcus pneumoniae* (3), *Moraxella catarrhalis* (1), *Pseudomonas aeruginosa* (1) and *Aspergillus* sp. (1). Bronchoscopy was repeated during an exacerbation. Defined as 2 of the 3 cardinal symptoms mentioned above, the number of patients with positive PSB, increased to 15 of 29 (51.7%), and included *H. influenzae (10)*, *S. pneumoniae* (3), *P. aeruginosa* (2) and *M. catarrhalis* (2). The same pathogens were isolated during chronic colonisation and during exacerbations, but it is very important to note that higher bacterial concentrations were found during exacerbations. It was suggested, by this study and by others, that the pathogen involved in colonisation was also that causing exacerbations.

COPD of the airway can be thought of as a test tube (Fig. 1). Certain patients have some bacteria within their airways on a long-term basis. This represents a balance in which the host defences contain the bacterial numbers but are not able to eradicate them. When an exacerbation occurs, the balance is upset and the microbial load increases, which attracts an inflammatory response and leads to cardinal Anthonisen-defined symptoms. The balance is probably more often upset because of further impairment of the host defences e.g. following a viral infection which allows the bacterium to increase in numbers, rather than a more virulent bacterial infection or infection by a strain that is not recognised by the host's immune defences.

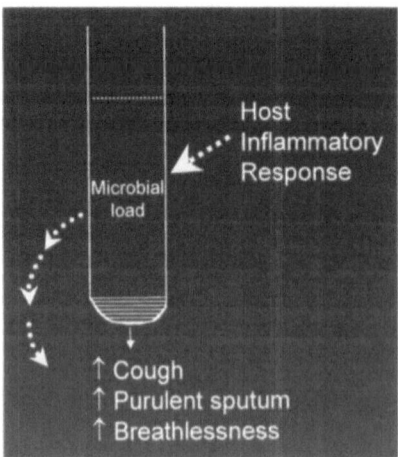

Fig. 1
Test tube model of bacterial bronchial infection

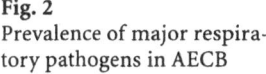

Fig. 2
Prevalence of major respiratory pathogens in AECB

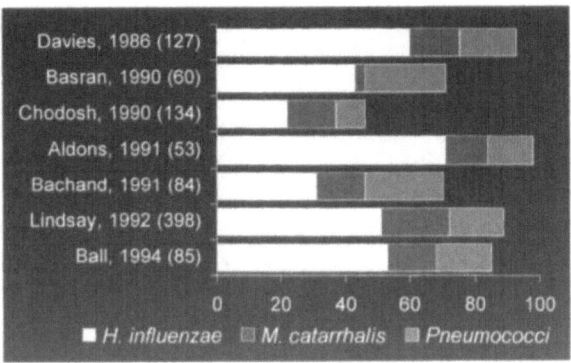

A number of studies (Fig. 2) [4] have demonstrated that the major pathogens in AECB are non-typable *H. influenzae* (30–70%), *M. catarrhalis* (10–20%) and *S. pneumoniae* (10–15%). Other species are sometimes isolated e.g. *Haemophilus parainfluenzae*, but their pathogenic role is less certain. Several recent studies have noted the increased importance of Gram-negative bacteria, e.g. *P. aeruginosa* in patients with severe airflow obstruction[5].

In recently published data[6], looking at factors associated with death in COPD, highly significant correlations were made with more severe airflow obstruction, patients who smoked more cigarettes through their lives, patients who were losing weight, and patients who were coughing up phlegm on a daily basis. However, only chronic mucus hypersecretion predicted death from an infectious cause. Chronic bronchitis is common in middle aged smokers in whom the prognosis is poor: 10 year mortality rising to 60% in comparison to 15% in non-smoking atopic controls. Mortality is highest in patients over 65.

Patients who have experienced 4 episodes in the last year or have a comedical condition, such as cardiovascular disease, have an increased risk of failure when they present with an exacerbation [2]. Older patients with a long history of chronic bronchitis who have a more severe airflow obstruction and who require systemic corticosteroids are also at greater risk [7, 8].

St. George's Respiratory Questionnaire is a quality of life measurement tool for the assessment of patients with COPD. A score is assigned to a patient based on 3 components: symptoms, activity and impact on daily life and general well being. A high score reflects a poor quality of life. Patients presenting with an ineffective exacerbation of COPD were questioned on enrolment and at weekly intervals and baseline values (full recovery from the exacerbation) were only achieved after 3 to 6 weeks. This is a much longer period of impaired health than is usually appreciated.

The use of antimicrobial agents in the treatment of patients with AECB has been controversial. A meta-analysis (Fig. 3) [9] summarising 9 randomised, double blind, placebo controlled, trials showed that overall there was only a fairly small benefit for the antibiotic treated group. However, in a landmark study (Table 1) [1] in which exacerbations were differentiated based on the 3 cardinal symptoms of increased cough with sputum production, increased dyspnea and

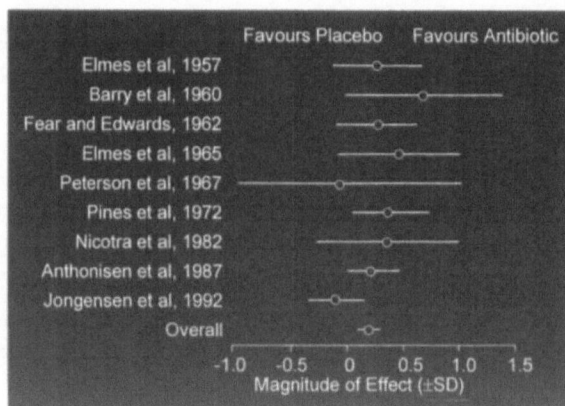

Fig. 3
Meta-analysis of placebo-controlled antibiotic trials in COPD

Table 1. Success of antimicrobial therapy in AECB

	Type I		Type II		Type III	
	active	placebo	active	placebo	active	placebo
Success	63	43	70	60	74	70
Failure/deterioration	34	53	26	37	23	30
Overall	Success:		antibiotic:	68%		
			placebo:	55%		
	Failure:		antibiotic:	10%		
			placebo:	19%		

sputum purulence, antibiotic therapy (amoxicillin, TMP/SMX and doxycycline) was associated with significant benefit, especially in patients classified as type 1 (all 3 symptoms), and to a lesser extent those classified as type 2 (2 symptoms). There was no difference in the use of antimicrobial therapy and placebo in patients classified as type 3 (one symptom).

Until the 1980s, antibiotics employed for the routine management of AECB were beta-lactams, macrolides, tetracyclines and cotrimoxazole. During the last 10 to15 years, susceptibility and resistance patterns of the commonly isolated pathogens has changed. The incidence of beta-lactamase production in non-typable *H. influenzae* has increased; ampicillin resistance has been demonstrated in some beta-lactamase negative *H. influenzae* and resistance to amoxicillin/clavulanic acid was found in a few beta-lactamase positive strains. Beta-lactamase production in *M. catarrhalis* is about 95%, pneumococcal penicillin resistance has risen dramatically, and penicillin resistant strains often demonstrate cross resistance with other antimicrobials such as the cephalosporins, macrolides, tetracyclines and TMP/SMX.

The goals of antimicrobial therapy are prompt response to acute infection so that the inflammatory response is suppressed and the patient is less likely to have further complications. An ideal antimicrobial agent must penetrate well into bronchial tissue, have a high sputum and tissue concentration/MIC ratio, should provide a long infection free interval, must have excellent in-vitro activity against the most frequent pathogens, have an acceptable toxicity profile, convenient dosage schedule and be cost effective. It must also have activity against beta-lactamase producing *H. influenzae* and *M. catarrhalis* and multi-drug resistant *S. pneumoniae*.

Therapy for AECB has been classified as first-line (ampicillin, amoxicillin, TMP/SMX, doxycycline) or second-line (cephalosporins, fluoroquinolones, extended spectrum macrolides/azalides, beta-lactam/beta-lactamase inhibitor combinations (amoxicillin/clavulanate).

Amoxicillin remains a very useful antibiotic in areas of low resistance. Oral cephalosporins have poor bioavailability. Clarithromycin has good activity against *S. pneumoniae* and *M. catarrhalis,* but poor activity against *H.influenzae* leading to poor eradication rates [10]. TMP/SMX resistance is more common now and it has an adverse side effect profile.

Fluoroquinolones have good but differing activity against pneumococci. Compared to ciprofloxacin and ofloxacin, the newer fluoroquinolones (e.g. moxifloxacin, trovafloxacin) have enhanced activity and all have excellent activity against beta-lactamase producing *M. catarrhalis* and *H. influenzae.* Fluoroquinolones concentrate in the bronchial mucosa at concentrations above the serum levels and the tissue penetration ratio is excellent. Data suggest an excellent early response, low rates of early relapse [10], a prolonged infection free interval (ciprofloxacin is 146 days) [11] and an established low level of toxicity.

Conclusion

Future investigations to establish the superiority of new antimicrobial agents may benefit from data collected using enhanced bacteriological techniques (e.g. PSB) and from studying their efficacy in sicker patients (Anthonisen type 1), and patients with risk factors for poor outcome and comorbidities. Also investigating the speed of resolution of symptoms, applying quality of life questionnaires and measuring exacerbation free intervals would be beneficial. Enrolment of patients prospectively would ensure the opportunity to enrich for patients with more advanced disease and to establish baseline data with which to compare exacerbation data and speed of return to baseline.

References

1. Anthonisen NR, Manfreda J, Warren CP, Hershfield ES, Harding GK, Nelson NA (1987) Antibiotic therapy in exacerbations of chronic obstructive pulmonary disease. Ann Intern Med 106:196–204
2. Ball P, Harris JM, Lawson D et al. (1995) Acute infective exacerbations of chronic bronchitis QJ Med 88:61–68
3. Monso E, Ruiz, J, Rosell, A, Manterola, J, Fiz, J, Morera, J, Ausina, V (1995) Bacterial infection in chronic obstructive pulmonary disease. A study of stable and exacerbated outpatients using the protected specimen brush. Am J Respir Crit Care Med 152:1316–1320

4. Ball P (1995) Epidemiology and treatment of chronic bronchitis and its exacerbations. Chest 108:43S–52S
5. Eller J, Ede A, Schaberg et al. (1998) Infective exacerbations of chronic bronchitis: relation between bacteriologic aetiology and lung function. Chest 113(6):1542–1548
6. Prescott E, Lange P, Vestbo J (1995) Chronic mucus hypersecretion in COPD and death from pulmonary infection. Europ Resp J 8:1333–1338
7. Grossman RF (1998) The value of antibiotics and the outcomes of antibiotic therapy of COPD. Chest 113:249S–255S
8. Wilson R (1995) Outcome predictors of bronchitis. Chest, 108:53 suppl–57 suppl
9. Saint S, Bent S, Vittinghoff E, Grady D (1995) Antibiotics in chronic obstructive pulmonary disease exacerbations. A meta-analysis. JAMA 273:957–960
10. Wilson R, Kubin R, Ballin I et al. (1999) Five day moxifloxacin therapy compared to seven day clarithromycin therapy for the treatment of acture exacerbations of chronic bronchitis. ECCMID JAC, in press
11. Chodosh S, McCarty J, Farkas S, Drehobi M, Tosiella R, Shan M et al. (1998) Randomized double-blind study of ciprofloxacin and cefuroxime axetil for treatment of acute bacterial exacerbations of chronic bronchitis. The Bronchitis Study Group. Clin Infect Dis 27(4): 722–729

Clinical Needs in the Millennium – Acute Exacerbations of Chronic Bronchitis – The Role of Moxifloxacin

30

DEBORAH CHURCH

Abstract. Four clinical studies were conducted in patients with AECB. Moxifloxacin (400 mg qd 5 or 10 d) was compared to cefuroxime (250 mg bid 10 days) and clarithromycin (500 mg bid 7/10 d). Clinical success with moxifloxacin (400 mg qd 5 d) was 89%, similar to comparators (87% and 89% respectively). Bacteriological success at day 17–24 post therapy was 87%.

Other fluoroquinolone comparative trials have demonstrated lower clinical success rates: levofloxacin (500 mg 7/10 d) 54% at day 21–28 and grepafloxacin (600 mg 10 d) 81% at day 14–28.

Introduction

Haemophilus influenzae is the most common etiological agent associated with acute exacerbations of chronic bronchitis (AECB). Moxifloxacin is 30–40% of infections highly active against *H. influenzae* (MIC_{90} 0.06 µg/mL) and also shows excellent in-vitro activity against the other major pathogens, *Moraxella catarrhalis* (0.06 µg/mL), *Streptococcus pneumoniae* (0.12–0.25 µg/mL), and minor pathogens, *Haemophilus parainfluenzae* (0.25 µg/mL), *Staphylococcus aureus* (0.12 µg/mL), *Escherichia coli* (0.006 µg/mL), *and Klebsiella pneumoniae* (0.25 µg/mL) [1–3].

Results and Discussion

The role of moxifloxacin in the treatment of acute exacerbations of chronic bronchitis (AECB) has been investigated in four clinical studies, one phase II and three phase III comparative, double blind, registration studies using FDA and IDSA guidelines. These studies involved over 2000 patients who were treated with moxifloxacin.

Enrolment criteria included a history of chronic bronchitis defined as a persistent cough and excessive secretion of mucus on most days for at least 3 consecutive months over 2 consecutive years (WHO definition). Anthonisen criteria were also applied in terms of defining the severity of the disease and included increased sputum volume, increased sputum purulence and increased breathlessness. Patients with all three parameters were classified as type I; two of three symptoms, as type II; and any one of the three plus cough or a range of minor symptoms, as type III.

The first study (106) was a phase II study to compare 200 mg and 400 mg moxifloxacin once daily with 400mg cefixime once daily for a minimum of 6 days and a maximum of 14 days in the treatment of patients of Anthonisen criteria severity type I and II. Study 124 was a phase III study, outside North America, to compare 400 mg moxifloxacin once daily for 5 days with 500 mg clarithromycin twice daily for 7 days in patients of severity type I and II. Study 127 was a phase III study in which the optimal dose of 400 mg moxifloxacin once daily for 2 durations of therapy of 5 or 10 days was compared to 500 mg clarithromycin twice daily for 10 days in patients of severity type I, II and III. Study 128 was a phase III study in which 200 mg and 400 mg moxifloxacin once daily was compared to 500 mg cefuroxime twice daily for a total of 10 days in patients of severity type I, II and III. Both studies 127 and 128 were carried out in North America and the majority of patients were of severity type I.

Clinical success rates (the test of cure) in the treatment of AECB are presented in Table 1. In study 128, a similar clinical success rate was achieved in patients treated with either 200 mg or 400 mg of moxifloxacin once daily for 10. Both had a higher clinical success rate than the comparator, 500 mg cefuroxime, twice daily for 10 days (87%).

In study 127, the clinical success rate of 400 mg moxifloxacin once daily for 10 days (91%) was slightly greater but not significantly different than the same dosage for 5 days, (89%), which was identical to the clinical success rate of 500 mg clarithromycin, twice daily for 10 days (89%). Study 124 demonstrated an identical clinical success rate for 400 mg moxifloxacin once daily for 5 days (89%) as in study 127, and a similar clinical success rate to that of the comparator, 500 mg clarithromycin twice daily for 7 days, which was also comparable to that of the same dosage for 10 days (88%).

The bacteriological success (test of cure) data is presented in Table 2. In study 128, a similar bacteriological success rate was achieved in patients treated with

Table 1. The clinical success rates in patients with acute exacerbations of chronic bronchitis (AECB) who were treated with either moxifloxacin or clarithromycin or cefuroxime

Study #	Moxifloxacin			Clarithromycin	Cefuroxime
	200 mg	400 mg			
	10 d	5 d	10 d		
124		287/322 (89)	–	289/327 (88)	–
127		222/250 (89)	234/256 (91)	224/251 (89)	–
128	161/170 (93)	–	157/170 (92)		161/185 (87)
Overall	(91)	509/572 (89)	391/426 (92)	513/578 (89)	161/185 (87)

% in parenthesis.

Table 2. The bacteriological success rate in patients with acute exacerbations of chronic bronchitis (AECB) who were treated with either moxifloxacin or clarithromycin or cefuroxime

	Moxifloxacin			Clarithromycin	Cefuroxime
	200 mg	400 mg			
	10 d	5 d	10 d		
124	–	98/115 (77)	–	71/114 (62)	–
127	–	127/143 (89)	135/148 (91)	110/129 (85)	–
128	72/77 (93)	–	67/73 (92)	–	72/85 (85)
Overall	(93)	225/258 (87)	202/221 (91)	253/328 (77)	

% in parenthesis.

either 200 mg or 400 mg of moxifloxacin once daily for 10 days (93 % and 92 %, respectively). Each had a higher bacteriological success rate than the comparator, 500 mg cefuroxime, twice daily for 10 days (85 %). In study 127, the bacteriological success rate of 400 mg moxifloxacin once daily for 10 days (91 %), was similar to that of the same dosage for 5 days (89 %), and both were higher than the bacteriological success rate of the comparator, 500 mg clarithromycin, twice daily for 10 days (85 %). Study 124 demonstrated a lower bacteriological success rate for 400 mg moxifloxacin once daily for 5 days (77 %) than that in study 127. The bacteriological success rate of the comparator, 500 mg clarithromycin, twice daily for 7 days was lower (62 %) than moxifloxacin and lower

Table 3. The bacteriological success rates against *Haemophilus influenzae*, *Streptococcus pneumoniae* and *Moraxella catarrhalis* in patients with acute exacerbations of chronic bronchitis (AECB) who were treated with either moxifloxacin, clarithromycin or cefuroxime

	Moxifloxacin			Clarithromycin	Cefuroxime
	200 mg	400 mg			
	10 d	5 d	10 d		
H. influenzae	24/25	73/81 (90.1)	49/51 (96.1)	56/84 (64.3)	22/27
S. pneumoniae	8/9	48/54 (88.9)	25/26 (96.2)	56/59 (94.9)	8/9
M. catarrhalis	10/10	43/50 (86.0)	33/35 (94.3)	47/48 (97.9)	7/10

% in parenthesis.

than that of the same dosage for 10 days. The differences between studies may be a reflection of the severity and complexity of the patients enrolled.

The bacteriological success rate of the three target pathogens, *H. influenzae*, *S. pneumoniae* and *M. catarrhalis*, at day 17–24 are presented in Table 3. The overall bacteriological success rates of the comparators were lower for each of the regimen, in particular with clarithromycin against *H. influenzae* (64%) and cefuroxime against *M. catarrhalis* (70%).

A comparison of the clinical response data of other fluoroquinolones in the recent published literature demonstrates variability in the clinical response. A clinical response of 92% was achieved with 500 mg Q.D. levofloxacin at 5 to 7 days post therapy [4] compared to 79% at 5 to 14 days post therapy in a similar study at the same dose [5]. This was reduced to 54% at 21 to 28 days post therapy. A clinical success rate of 81% was achieved with grepafloxacin 14 to 28 days post therapy [6]. In comparison 5 days of 400 mg once daily moxifloxacin yielded clinical success rates of 89% at 17–24 days in almost 600 patients.

Conclusion

From clinical experience in the treatment of AECB, moxifloxacin has shown antibacterial activity against the key pathogens which corroborates in-vitro findings, including resistant strains. As it penetrates into bronchial mucosa in excess of the MIC values, this leads to clinical response rates of 89% and bacteriological response rates of 87% with 400 mg moxifloxacin given once daily after 5 days treatment.

References

1. Focht J (1998) In vitro activity of Bay 12-8039 compared with other fluoroquinolones against bacterial strains from upper and lower respiratory tract infections in general practice. Poster at ICID, Boston
2. Heisig P, Wiedemann B (1997) In vitro activity of the new 8-methoxyquinolone Bay 12-8039 against defined mutants of Escherichia coli and Staphylococcus aureus. Poster ICAAC, Toronto
3. Petersen U, Bremm KD, Dalhoff A et al. (1996) Synthesis and in vitro activity of Bay 12-8039, a new methoxyquinolone. Poster ICAAC, New Orleans
4. Habib MP, Gentry LO, Rodriguez-Gomez G, Morowitz W, Williams R (1996) A multicentre randomised study comparing the efficacy and safety of oral levofloxacin versus cefaclor in the treatment of acute bacterial exacerbations of chronic bronchitis. 36th ICAAC, New Orleans, USA
5. Shah PM, The international Study Group (1997) Levofloxacin versus cefuroxime axetil in the treatment of acute exacerbations of chronic bronchitis. 37th ICAAC Toronto Canada, 371 Abstr LM-38
6. Chodosh S, Lakshminarayan S, Swarz H, Breisch S (1998) Efficacy and safety of a 10 day course of 400 or 600 milligrams of grepafloxacin once daily for the treatment of acute bacterial exacerbations of chronic bronchitis: comparison with a 10 day course of 500 milligrams of ciprofloxacin twice daily. Antimicrob Agents Chem 42:1114–1120

CHAPTER 31

Clinical Needs in the Millennium – Rhinosinusitis 31

VALERIE J. LUND

Abstract. Acute infectious rhinosinusitis, both viral and bacterial, affects more than a billion persons annually and is the most common health complaint in the United States. Bacterial rhinosinusitis may be broadly divided into acute or chronic infection, the distinction being made in pathophysiology, microbiology, and symptomology. The bacteriological profile mirrors that in the lower respiratory tract and is subject to the same problems of antimicrobial resistance. A number of factors predispose individuals to the development of infection, most notable being impairment of mucociliary function. For acute infectious rhinosinusitis, a wide range of antibiotics are used first line, including broad-spectrum penicillins, cephalosporins and tetracyclines. There is also little consensus on the second-line antibiotics which might include those with beta-lactamase resistance to penicillins, macrolides or quinolones. A proportion of patients would undoubtedly improve without treatment, but meta-analysis confirms that antibiotics are significantly more effective than placebo in curing symptoms and may well diminish the progression to chronic disease or one of the severe life-threatening complications of acute infection.

Sinusitis or more appropriately, rhinosinusitis is defined as inflammation of the lining of the nose and paranasal sinuses and is characterised by one or more of the following symptoms: nasal congestion, rhinorrhoea, sneezing, itching and hyposmia.

The viral form of acute rhinosinusitis, the common cold, represents the most common health complaint in the western world; affecting 1 billion persons annually. Furthermore, 0.5–2% of viral upper respiratory tract infections are complicated by acute bacterial rhinosinusitis (ABRS) leading to about 20 million cases in the USA each year.

In terms of health impact, chronic rhinosinusitis is extremely important. In studies of quality of life, using instruments such as the SF 36, chronic rhinosinusitis has been shown to have an impact equivalent to conditions such as diabetes, rheumatoid arthritis and severe hypertension.

Controversy concerning the nature of infectious rhinosinusitis has resulted in considerable variation in classification and definition, and recent reviews have sought to rectify this [1]. Rhinosinusitis can be classified as acute, recurrent acute, chronic, acute on chronic or subacute (Fig. 1). In acute rhinosinusitis, inflammation and infection are of limited duration, clearing spontaneously or with appropriate therapy. Acute episodes can recur (recurrent acute) but normalisation of the mucosa occurs between episodes. Chronic rhinosinusitis may occur due to failure of therapy of an acute infection or it may develop without a recognised acute phase and is persistent. Many patients with chronic rhino-

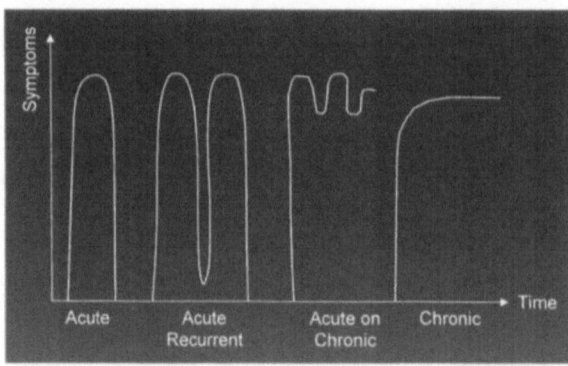

Fig. 1
Classification of acute and
chronic rhinosinusitis

sinusitis develop additional acute episodes of infection which resolve with treatment but the chronic condition remains with residual damage to the sinus mucosa.

The differentiation between acute and chronic rhinosinusitis is not simple. Consequently, duration of symptoms is used to distinguish between the two. Acute rhinosinusitis is classified as having symptoms for less than 4 weeks and chronic rhinosinusitis as having symptoms for greater than 12 weeks. In between the two conditions there is a period of time that is classified as subacute.

There are clear differences in pathophysiology between acute and chronic rhinosinusitis. Acute rhinosinusitis is an exudative process with necrosis, haemorrhage, ulceration and with neutrophil infiltrates; the chronic form is a proliferative process with fibrosis of the lamina propria and infiltration of lymphocytes, plasma cells and eosinophils.

Among patients with suspected ABRS, only about 60% have verification of the presence of bacteria by sinus aspirate culture. The dominant pathogens, in studies of sinus aspirates are *Streptococcus pneumoniae* (31%, range 20–35%) and *Haemophilus influenzae* (21%, 6–26%). Other pathogens implicated included anaerobes (6%, 0–8%), *Staphylococcus aureus* (4%, 0–8%), *Streptococcus pyogenes* (2%, 1–3%) and *Moraxella catarrhalis* (2%, 2–10%). The bacterial aetiology of chronic rhinosinusitis is less well studied than ABRS and results are not consistent. Pathogens have been classified into three groups (Table 1): group 1 includes pathogens implicated in acute rhinosinusitis and probably responsible for acute exacerbations of the infection; group 2 includes pathogens which may be important in conditions such as cystic fibrosis and group 3 includes other bacteria whose significance and role as pathogens is questionable.

There is a difference in the degree of symptomology between the acute and chronic situations. The major symptoms of ABRS in adults are facial pain or pressure, nasal congestion, nasal discharge and fever. Minor symptoms include cough, headache, halitosis and earache. Cough and purulent discharge are major factors and otitis media is a common coexisting condition in children with rhinosinusitis. Major symptoms of chronic rhinosinusitis are pain and pressure, obstruction, purulent discharge, hyposmia/ anosmia and non-asthmatic cough

Table 1
Bacterial aetiology of chronic rhinosinusitis

Group 1
- *S. pneumoniae, H. influenzae, M. catarrhalis*
- *S. intermedius*
- High titres from sinus aspirates
- Acute exacerbations or possibly on-going disease

Group 2
- *S. aureus, P. aeruginosa*
- Sinus aspirates in cystic fibrosis
- Post-operative sinus cavities, persistent infection
- Probable cause of disease

Group 3
- *S. epidermidis*, corynebacteria, anaerobes
- Low titres from swabs at surgery
- ? role as pathogens

(in children) and minor symptoms include fever, halitosis, fatigue, dental pain and cough (in adults). Fever is more of a feature of acute infection whereas a decreased sense of smell is common in chronic infection.

There are many aetiological factors that can be responsible for the development of infection including allergy; anatomical variations; immune deficiencies (AIDS); and mucociliary abnormalities (cystic fibrosis).

The pathogenesis of rhinosinusitis is incompletely understood but one of the most important factors may be mucociliary clearance mechanisms, which are largely responsible in health, for the elimination of an attacker, such as bacteria or viruses, occasionally with an acute controlled inflammatory response. Failure to eliminate an attacker may elicit a vicious circle of events that is difficult to break in which bacteria allow or facilitate damage to occur, to the mucociliary clearance mechanisms, which in turn leads to amplification of the inflammatory response and damage to the surrounding tissue (Fig. 2).

Fig. 2
Pathogenesis of rhinosinusitis

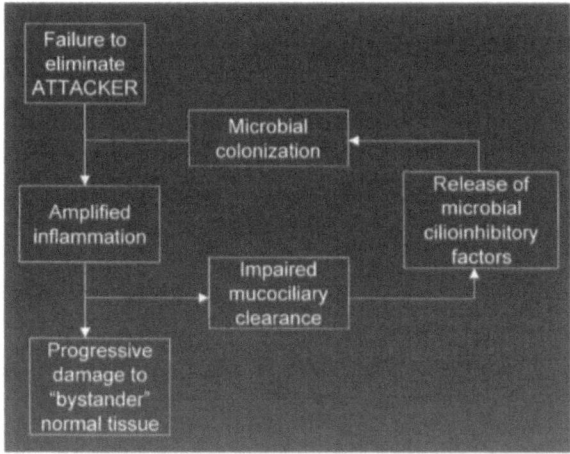

Viral upper respiratory infections commonly precede bacterial rhinosinusitis. Viruses implicated include picornaviruses (rhinovirus, Coxsackie virus, reovirus and echovirus), influenza, parainfluenza, adenovirus and respiratory syncytial virus. In studies of intranasal inoculation of non-immune volunteers with rhinovirus, initiation of infection is followed by stimulation of inflammatory pathways and the parasympathetic nervous system resulting in engorgement of capacitance vessels in the venous erectile tissue of the turbinates, extracellular leakage of plasma, discharge of seromucinous glands and goblet cells and neural stimulation leading to pain, sneezing and cough reflexes, the familiar symptoms of a cold. The sinus mucosa shows signs of oedema, goblet cell hyperplasia and epithelial desquamation. Nasal and sinus mucosal abnormalities have been identified on computed tomographic (CT) scans in almost 90% of subjects with confirmed colds caused by rhinoviruses [2]. In 77% of the patients there was evidence for infundibulum occlusion which resolved spontaneously in most patients, but in some a secondary bacterial infection developed. The secondary bacterial infection may be due to the marked interference or cessation of mucociliary function draining the sinus cavities and to ostiomeatal obstruction as evidenced by the increased viscosity of the secretion and slowing or paralysis of the cilia.

Commensal bacteria in the nose and nasopharynx are the same bacteria that cause ABRS. The factors that determine whether bacteria invade the normally sterile sinuses during viral rhinosinusitis are unknown, but sneezing, coughing, and nose blowing can exert pressure differentials, adequate enough for bacteria to enter and multiply in an obstructed sinus.

Experimental maxillary sinus infections in rabbits have demonstrated that *Haemophilus influenzae* and *Streptococcus pneumoniae* produce toxins that destroy ciliated epithelial cells and damage mucosal cells [3]. Recovery from the disease process requires regeneration of ciliated epithilium as well as relief of ostial obstruction. Studies of the effect of *S. pneumoniae* in nasal turbinate tissue organ cultures have demonstrated a 24% decrease (Table 2) in ciliary beat frequency compared to a control over a 24 h period [4]. *Pseudomonas aeruginosa* also inhibits ciliary action by the production of pyocyanin, 1-hydroxyphenazine and rhamnolipid.

Table 2. The effect of infection with *Streptococcus pneumoniae* on the ciliary beat frequency of nasal turbinate organ cultures

Time h	0	4	16	24
Experiments n	6	7	5	4
CBF Hz				
Control	11.1 (1.5)	10.3 (1.0)	10.1 (0.5)	9.6 (2.1)
Infected[a]	10.9 (1.2)	9.5 (1.8)	8.8 (1.3)	7.3 (1.3)
% ciliary slowing	2	8	13	24
P value[b]	ns	ns	<0.05	<0.01

[a] Mean, standard deviation in parenthesis.
[b] Wilcoxon Sign Rank Test.

Several studies have suggested that antibiotics play a controversial role in the treatment of ABRS [5–7]. In a meta analysis of clinical outcomes in 6 trials of 761 patients comparing antibiotics with placebo for treating uncomplicated acute sinusitis it was demonstrated that antibiotics decreased the incidence of clinical failures by half. However, over two thirds of the patients treated with placebo showed spontaneous resolution or improvement of symptoms. Treatment with newer more expensive antibiotics did not seem to reduce the rate of treatment failure beyond what amoxicillin and cotrimoxazole could achieve [8].

Initial antimicrobial treatment of acute rhinosinusitis is empirical. In a study of 40 million prescriptions from primary care physicians in USA and the countries of Western Europe, the commonest antibiotics prescribed for acute and chronic rhinosinusitis were amoxicillin, amoxicillin-clavulanate, cefuroxime axetil and clarithromycin. Antimicrobial resistance to respiratory pathogens, including multiple resistance among *S. pneumoniae* and beta-lactamase production by *H. influenzae* and *M. catarrhalis*, represents an increasingly important therapeutic problem. Many patients who fail treatment will go on to develop chronic infection or more rarely go on to develop some of the complications of acute bacterial rhinosinusitis including meningitis, brain abscess, orbital cellulitis and subdural empyema which may result in blindness and occasionally death. Thus, antimicrobials of choice should penetrate well and attain high concentrations in the infected sinus mucosa, have a broad spectrum of activity, are stable in the presence of beta-lactamases and are active against penicillin resistant pneumococci. These include second generation cephalosporins and fluoroquinolones. Fluoroquinolones provide good coverage for all four key rhinosinusitis pathogens (*S. pneumoniae, H. influenzae, M. catarrhalis* and *S. aureus*) as well as penicillin-resistant strains of *S. pneumoniae* and beta-lactamase producing strains of *H. influenzae, M. catarrhalis* and *S. aureus* and are effective when administered once daily [9].

References

1. International Rhinosinusitis Advisory Board (1997) Infectious rhinosinusitis in adults: classification, etiology and management. ENT Journal 76 (suppl) 12:1–22
2. Gwaltney JM Jr. (1996) Acute community acquired sinusitis. Clin Infect Dis 23:1209–1223
3. Hinni ML, McCaffrey TV, Kasperbauer JL (1992) Early mucosal changes in experimental sinusitis. Otolaryngol Head Neck Surgery 107:537–548
4. Feldman C, Read R, Rutman A, Jeffery PK et al. (1992) The interaction of Streptococcus pneumoniae with intact human respiratory mucosa in vitro. Eur Resp J 5(5):576–583
5. Huck W, Reed BD, Nelson RW et al. (1993) Cefaclor vs amoxicillin in the treatment of acute recurrent and chronic sinusitis. Arch Fam Med 2:497
6. Lindbaek M, Hjortdahl P, Johnsen UL (1996) Randomized double blind placebo controlled trial of penicillin V and amoxicillin in treatment of acute sinus infections in adults. BMJ 313:325
7. Haye R, Lingaas E., Holvik HO et al. (1996) Efficacy and safety of azithromycin vs. phenoxymethylpenicillin in the treatment of acute maxillary sinusitis. Eur J Clin Microbial Infect Dis 15:849
8. De Ferranti SD, Ioannidis JPA, Lau J, Anninger WV, Barza M (1998) Are amoxicillin and folate inhibitors as effective as other antibiotics for acute sinusitis? A meta-analysis. BMJ 317:632–637
9. Proctor RA, Bartlett JG (1997) Respiratory Infections in the year 2000: Managing Rhinosinusitis. Proceedings of the consensus conference sponsored by the University of Wisconsin Medical School and School of Pharmacy, p 1–24

Chapter 32

Clinical Needs in the Millienium – Rhinosinusitis – The Role of Moxifloxacin

Barbara Hampel

Abstract. Four clinical trials were conducted in North America and Europe with patients suffering from acute sinusitis. Moxifloxacin (400 mg qd 7/10 d) was compared to cefuroxime (250 mg bid 10 d). Clinical results were comparable (92.6 % vs. 92.8 % respectively); however bacteriological response was higher among patients receiving moxifloxacin treatment for 7 days (95.6 %) and 10 days (98 %) vs. those receiving cefuroxime treatment (87.7 %). Eradication of *S. pneumoniae* was achieved in 98.6 % of cultures from patients treated with 400 mg moxifloxacin for 7 days, 95 % from patients treated for 10 days and 96 % from patients treated with cefuroxime. Eradication of *H. influenzae* was 98 %, 100 % and 88 %, respectively, and eradication of *M. catarrhalis* was 94 %, 100 % and 93 %, respectively.

Introduction

Streptococcus pneumoniae is the most common etiological agent associated with rhinosinusitis. Moxifloxacin is highly active against clinical isolates of *S. pneumoniae* (MIC_{90} 0.12 – 0.25 µg/mL) collected worldwide [1]. Moxifloxacin also shows excellent in vitro activity against other pathogens associated with rhinosinusitis including *Haemophilus influenzae* (MIC_{90} 0.06 µg/mL), *Staphylococcus aureus* (0.12 µg/mL), *Streptococcus pyogenes* (0.25 µg/mL), *Moraxella catarrhalis* (0.06 µg/mL) and anaerobes. In an investigation of 180 anaerobic pulmonary isolates including *Bacteroides* spp., *Prevotella* spp., *Fusobacterium* spp., *Clostridium* spp., *Peptostreptococcus* spp., and nonspore forming Gram-positive rods, only one isolate was resistant to moxifloxacin, a *Clostridium* spp. (MIC_{90} 8 µg/mL). The rest had MIC values ≤1 µg/mL [2, 3].

Results and Discussion

The role of moxifloxacin in the treatment of acute rhinosinusitis has been investigated in four clinical studies; 3 randomised, double blind, phase III trials, and one uncontrolled trial.

Enrolment criteria included suspected acute maxillary rhinosinusitis as suggested by paranasal sinus X-ray (Water's view) to confirm the diagnosis and at least two of the following criteria: nasal congestion, post-nasal drainage, cough or throat clearing, frontal headache, molar tenderness or pain, or prevalent nasal discharge. Acute sinusitis was defined as signs or symptoms that were present for less than or equal to 4 weeks with no more than 2 episodes in the previous year.

The primary efficacy parameter in all of the studies was either the clinical response at the first post treatment visit (the European approach) or the overall clinical response at follow-up carrying forward clinical failures (the American approach). Collection of material for bacteriological assessment was carried out by sinus puncture (USA, Europe), cannulation (France) and swab (Europe).

Study 125 was an uncontrolled study in USA of 400 mg moxifloxacin once daily for 7 days in 324 patients. Study 116 was a randomised double blind phase III study in Europe to compare 400 mg moxifloxacin once daily for 7 days with 250 mg cefuroxime axetil twice daily for 10 days in the treatment of acute rhinosinusitis in 436 patients. Study 126 was a randomised double blind phase III study in North America to compare 400 mg moxifloxacin once daily for 7 days with 250 mg cefuroxime axetil twice daily for 10 days in the treatment of acute rhinosinusitis in 373 patients. Study 161 was a randomised double blind phase III study in Europe to compare 400 mg moxifloxacin once daily for 10 days with 250 mg cefuroxime axetil twice daily for 10 days in 439 patients.

In study 125, clinical resolution was achieved in 301/324 (92.9%) patients treated with 400 mg moxifloxacin once daily for 7 days. In the first of the phase III studies, study 126, clinical resolution was achieved in 162/186 (87.1%) patients treated with 400 mg moxifloxacin once daily for 7 days compared to 174/187 (93.1%) patients treated with 250 mg cefuroxime axetil twice daily for 10 days. In the second phase III study, 116, clinical resolution was achieved in 204/211 moxifloxacin (96.7%) and 204/225 cefuroxime axetil (90.7%) patients, respectively. In the third, study 161, clinical resolution was achieved in 203/217 (93.5%) patients treated with 400 mg moxifloxacin once daily for 10 days compared to 210/222 (94.6%) patients treated with 250 mg cefuroxime axetil twice daily for 10 days. The overall clinical response (Table 1) was similar in each of the treatment groups (92.5% moxifloxacin vs. 92.8% cefuroxime).

Bacteriological resolution was higher in those patients treated with moxifloxacin than with cefuroxime. In study 125, bacteriological resolution was achieved in 72/74 (97%) patients treated with 400mg moxifloxacin once daily for

Table 1. The clinical resolution of acute rhinosinusitis in patients treated with either moxifloxacin, 7 or 10 days, or cefuroxime

Clinical resolution (%) at test-of-cure-visit		
Study	Moxifloxacin[a]	Cefuroxime[b]
125 (USA)	301/324 (92.9)	–
126 (NA)	162/186 (87.1)	174/187 (93.1)
116 (EU)	204/211 (96.7)	204/225 (90.7)
161 (EU)	203/217 (93.5)[c]	210/222 (94.6)
Overall	667/721 (92.6)	588/634 (92.8)

[a] 400 mg qd 7 days.
[b] 250 mg bid 10 days.
[c] 400 mg qd 10 days.

Table 2. The bacteriological resolution of acute sinusitis in patients treated with either moxifloxacin, 7 or 10 days, or cefuroxime

Bacteriological resolution (%) at test-of-cure-visit			
Study	Moxi 7	Moxi 10	Cefuroxime
125	72/74 (97)	–	–
116	103/109 (94)	–	96/115 (83)
161		84/86 (98)	68/72 (94)
Overall	175/183 (95.6)	84/86 (98)	164/187 (87.7)

7 days. In study 116, bacteriological resolution was achieved in 103/109 (94%) patients treated with 400 mg moxifloxacin once daily for 7 days compared to 96/115 (83%) patients treated with 250 mg cefuroxime axetil twice daily for 10 days. In study 161, bacteriological resolution was achieved in 84/86 (98%) patients treated with 400 mg moxifloxacin for 10 days compared to 68/72 (94%) patients treated with 250 mg cefuroxime axetil twice daily for 10 days. The overall bacteriological response rate (Table 2) was greater for patients treated with 400 mg moxifloxacin for 10 days (98%) than those treated with 400 mg moxifloxacin for 7 days (95.6%), but both were greater than for patients treated with cefuroxime axetil for 10 days (87.7%).

It should be noted that the bacteriological samples were obtained by different techniques. Study 125 used sinus puncture, which is the most invasive, and at this time the only method approved by the FDA. The other studies used several methodologies, sinus puncture, cannulation and swabs. The different methods of collection of material for bacteriological assessment did not have any effect on the rate of isolation or the type of pathogen cultured. The predominant pathogens were *S. pneumoniae*, *H. influenzae* and *M. catarrhalis* (Table 3). A high incidence of positive bacteriological cultures (52%) was achieved in the European studies. The eradication rates were similar in all the studies. Eradication of *S. pneumoniae* was achieved in 98.6% of cultures from patients treated with 400 mg moxifloxacin for 7 days, 95% from patients treated for 10 days and 96% from patients treated with cefuroxime. Eradication of *H. influenzae* was 98%,

Table 3. The bacteriological resolution of specific pathogens in acute sinusitis in patients treated with either moxifloxacin, 7 or 10 days, or cefuroxime

Accumulated bacteriological success (%) post-treatment			
Organism	Moxi 7	Moxi 10	Cefuroxime
S. pneumoniae	68/69 (98.6)	36/38 (95)	77/80 (96)
H. influenzae	58/59 (98)	17/17 (100)	45/51 (88)
M. catarrhalis	30/32 (94)	10/10 (100)	13/14 (93)

N.B. There was no difference in the frequency or type of organism isolated by either sinus puncture or endoscopy.

100 % and 88 %, respectively, and eradication of *M. catarrhalis* was 94 %, 100 % and 93 %, respectively.

Conclusion

Moxifloxacin has excellent in-vitro and in-vivo antibacterial activity against the key pathogens associated with rhinosinusitis and kills them rapidly. It penetrates into the sinuses considerably in excess of the MIC values and it achieves an overall clinical response of 92.5 % with a bacteriological response of 98 % following treatment with 400 mg moxifloxacin once daily for 7 – 10 days.

It can be concluded from these data that 400 mg moxifloxacin once daily shows greater clinical and bacteriological efficacy than 250 mg cefuroxime axetil twice daily for 10 days in the treatment of acute rhinosinusitis, and that 400 mg moxifloxacin given once daily for 7 days is as efficacious as given for 10 days.

References

1. Dalhoff A (1998) Moxifloxacin – Review of Microbiology. Antipneumococcal activity. Poster at New Quinolone Symposium, Denver
2. Focht J (1998) In vitro activity of Bay 12-8039 compared with other flouroquinolones against bacterial strains from upper and lower respiratory tract infections in general practice. Poster ICID, Boston
3. Wexler HM, Molitoris E, Finegold SM (1998) In vitro activity of moxifloxacin against bacteria isolated from pulmonary specimens. Poster ICAAC, San Diego

CHAPTER 33

Discussion on Clinical Needs in the Millennium 33

G. Hoffken: We have heard excellent presentations from our speakers and we now have time for questions. Moxifloxacin has demonstrated excellent clinical results. That is one part of the picture. The other part is the place of this drug in treating patients with these kinds of infections. Which patients need this drug? We have to define the patients.

Professor Léophonte, what is the place for moxifloxacin in community acquired pneumonia?

P. Léophonte: It is a very difficult question. You see different guidelines in different European countries, and not all fluoroquinolones were included, or sometimes were in association with another antibiotic in place of a macrolide. The problem now is: do we initially treat all the community acquired pneumonia with moxifloxacin because it is active against the main pathogens? I am not sure it would be a good solution because we may have some problems like the development of resistance. I think today it is not for the first line treatment of patients without risk, but it may be a second line treatment in patients after failure of the first treatment or those patients with risk factors. Currently, these prescriptions are for a beta-lactam and a macrolide; these are the cases I think would be a good indication for moxifloxacin alone.

QUESTION: In the U.S. it is suggested that certain classes of antibiotics are no longer used and that the susceptibility of *H. influenzae* or *S. pneumoniae* to quinolones is better than with cephalosporins or macrolides. For example, it was mentioned that the MIC values for clarithromycin against several strains was more than 8 mg/mL, but the clinical outcomes were not given. Did the strains with the high MIC values to clarithromycin come from patients who were treatment failures? What we want to know is if the microbiology data correlate with clinical outcomes. The correlation does not appear to be there at present. In spite of the microbiology data, such as high MIC values, clarithromycin is still a good drug.

M. Springsklee: You are right. We do not have sufficient treatment failures to draw a conclusion at this point. However, with sicker patients in ongoing studies, I am sure that the differences we would expect from the in-vitro and pharmacodynamic profile of moxifloxacin will be clearer.

QUESTION: The French have enormous resistance problems but for us, in Italy, the major problem is *H. influenzae* and its resistance to macrolides. For me, an antibiotic with such characteristics as moxifloxacin could be a first choice. Do you agree?

P. Léophonte: Yes. In France we have a certain level of resistance. The majority of the pneumococcal strains had MIC values greater than 2 mg/L, but with 3 g of amoxicillin we can treat the patients. The problem for us in the patients without risk is they may be increasing the resistance of pneumococcus. In cases where we want to broaden the spectrum of the treatment, it would be interesting to try a single antibiotic, like moxifloxacin, instead of the combination of a beta-lactam and a macrolide.

L. Mandell: I agree with Professor Léophonte. The concern with the IDSA guide-lines was that outpatients were one big group and they listed macrolides, quino-lones and doxycycline. Depending on how you interpret it, it could mean fluoro-quinolones for everything, which I think is wrong. The updated ATS guidelines and the currently updated Canadian and Canadian Thoracic Society guidelines will stay with the split in the outpatients. Some outpatients are relatively young and certainly some are quite healthy without risk factors and, despite the evi-dence for increasing MIC values to macrolides, there is no evidence of treatment failures. We will put the quinolones at risk as a class if we start using them in all those patients. The feeling is to continue with macrolides. If you had an out-patient who fits the Fine class I and II criteria, who does not require admission to hospital, has a structural lung disease, recently had antibiotics or steroids, that person would benefit from a fluoroquinolone. Also, the group that is admitted to hospital would benefit from a quinolone because there the standard would be beta-lactam and macrolide. The quinolone allows you to give one drug instead of two so it is logistically easier and cheaper. There is also a functional benefit in elderly patients who can be treated with an oral agent and maintain their mobility. I think the quinolones definitely have a tremendous role to play; they should not be used in all cases and that will ensure that the class is around for longer.

QUESTION: Concerning AECB, perhaps it is time to review the so-called Anthonisen criteria. For example, if cough is to be in the definition of chronic bronchitis, the Anthonisen criteria do not consider cough. There is no considera-tion for wheezes and rales. We have to define better markers then measure these markers. It is also necessary to define criteria for the effect of new drugs. The well-defined drug study of Anthonisen showed a 67% improvement which is not the 95% being claimed for new drugs. Is this because the previous criteria were insufficient or that new drugs are better than the doxycyclines?

ANSWER: To defend Anthonisen's study, it is very easy to apply the grading. General practitioners had never heard of Nick Anthonisen or the grading, but the patients they considered to be at risk, more seriously ill and requiring an antibiotic, they pick the Anthonisen criteria. General practitioners who are dealing with these patients many times a day, have worked with the Anthonisen definitions independently.

I would agree that we should develop other markers of bacterial involvement. For future antibiotic trials in this area, quality of life questionnaires, speed of recovery and simplified pharmacoeconomic data are going to be the results that differentiate superiority of the new agents.

Part 5
Round Table Discussion

CHAPTER 34

Round Table Discussion – Introduction   **34**

C. Carbon: I want to introduce the round table discussion by highlighting some issues.

What is our role as infectious disease and microbiology experts in the development of newer antimicrobials? It is to validate preclinical information by defining clinical efficacy through well-designed trials. It is also to define clinical indications for a new drug that demonstrates its efficacy, efficiency and cost effectiveness.

Is resistance a clinical manifestation of microbial promiscuity or vice versa? It is necessary to consider not only efficacy but also the short-term effects on the patient. It is necessary to realise that under-dosing and length of treatment have an influence on the selection of resistant mutants. Are there weapons to slow resistance? There are with the newer quinolones, provided proper doses and dose regimens are used.

Should hospital and community acquired respiratory infections be separated or are they a continuum? This is an important question that will be addressed by the two panels. There are similarities such as the optimal use of antibiotics and the interpretation of failure. Perhaps the differences are the severity of the cases, the patient's environment and the technical facilities available to the physician.

Can we assimilate all these new data and provide appropriate messages to fellow prescribers? We can and there are two main messages; use new compounds for validated indications and avoid under-dosing.

CHAPTER 35

Round Table Discussion – Hospital Issues　　35

D. Talan: As clinicians we must take what we have learned about moxifloxacin and consider how we will integrate this drug into our management of infected patients. Here we have an expert panel which will address treatment issues for patients who have infections serious enough to bring them into the hospital.

What is the role of moxifloxacin either for intra-abdominal infections due to a ruptured appendix or for the complicated surgical patient, who has had multiple operations, has an intra-abdominal abscess and has had several courses of antimicrobial therapy?

S. Gorbach: I believe that moxifloxacin, in an iv form, would be a good drug for secondary peritonitis. The more complicated forms, e. g. tertiary peritonitis, involve resistant organisms. This drug might be a suitable candidate in mixed therapy of these complicated infections.

Its advantages are the range of activity, the penetration into tissue and the aminoglycoside sparing effect. That is we do not use a drug that may produce renal damage. I am interested in more microbiological data and animal studies in intra-abdominal infections, but I hope to see this drug used for this indication.

D. Talan: Would this drug have the potential for therapy in pelvic infections in women, whether it be pelvic inflammatory disease and salpingitis or endometritis?

J. Turnidge: There is the potential for a very interesting role for moxifloxacin for this condition. In addition to the poly-microbial nature of the intra-abdominal sepsis complicating pelvic inflammatory disease, the physician also has to cure the gonococcus, chlamydia and possibly mycoplasmas. There are many guidelines with poly-antimicrobial solutions to the polymicrobial problems, but not many women can tolerate the therapies. If the drug covers all these organisms, it will be the future solution for this condition and turn it into an outpatient disease.

D. Talan: Can we now consider a more specialised problem, that is the neutropenic or cancer patient with fever? Fluoroquinolones have been used for prophylaxis and treatment. Consideration is being given to stratifying low risk patients for outpatient oral therapy. What is the role for moxifloxacin in this special patient population?

R. Garraffo: I have no easy answer to a difficult question since the use of fluoroquinolones in febrile neutropenic patients may lead to selection of resistant Gram-positive cocci, especially with older agents. Moxifloxacin has a better antibacterial spectrum, especially against staphylococci and streptococci. It has low MIC values and good activity against previous fluoroquinolone-resistant strains. It has good pharmacodynamic and good pharmacokinetic properties, especially rapid tissue penetration not modified by the neutropenic state. Moxifloxacin is well tolerated and has a lack of pharmacological interaction.

These are all advantages which could lead to reconsidering the role of fluoroquinolones in febrile neutropenic patients. Although, I would be cautious regarding selection of resistant strains such as *Pseudomonas aeruginosa* at current dosing.

D. Talan: I think we accept that moxifloxacin is an ideal drug for the seriously ill pneumonia patient. Could it be used as empirical treatment for nosocomial acquired pneumonia? In this indication there are resistant organisms, *Legionella,* and a significant number caused by pneumococcus. So, where does moxifloxacin fit in treatment of nosocomial pneumonia?

G. San Pedro: The data that we have seen certainly speaks to its activity against those organisms. I would like to see more data from a study on nosocomial pneumonia, but the indications are that moxifloxacin will be a good drug.

D. Talan: We face a number of problems with chronic mixed infections of soft tissues and bones, particularly in diabetes with osteomyelitis or chronic foot infections. What is the potential role for this drug for empirical therapy for these types of infections?

A. Rodloff: We have some experience with fluoroquinolones with diabetic foot infections where they have been used, although not as monotherapy. There is a mixed infection with staphylococci, other Gram-positives, a multitude of Gram-negatives and anaerobic bacteria. The anaerobes may impair the immunofunction of the host so they play a role and complicate these infections. Moxifloxacin may not be the ideal agent because *Pseudomonas* spp. play a role (but we await studies) and, despite the good pharmacokinetics, the activity against this organism is insufficient. However, for the other organisms it is positively a good choice.

D. Talan: What about the problems of community acquired pneumonia (CAP) and the hospitalised patients? We are all aware of the mounting resistance of pneumococci to macrolides. Yet I am impressed with the popularity, in the U.S., of these therapies, especially azithromycin and clarithromycin. Dr. Leeper, have you any comments on this paradox?

K. Leeper: Macrolides are one of the antimicrobial classes most frequently prescribed for treating CAP; they have been sanctioned by the ATS and the IDSA. There has been an increase in penicillin-resistant pneumococci coupled with an increase in macrolide-resistant pneumococci. At least three cases were reported last year in which there appeared to be treatment failures as a result of macrolides being used initially for treatment of CAP. In-vitro activity of any antimicrobial agent does not necessarily translate into clinical outcome.

I had personal experience of a paediatric patient who was treated initially with azithromycin for a lower respiratory tract infection. The patient did not respond, became very sick and probably should have been hospitalised with fluids and an appropriate antibiotic. However, she was successfully treated with a quinolone, illustrating that CAP patients can be treated in this manner.

D. Talan: If we see macrolides and quinolones become more frequently prescribed, will we see increasing MIC values then actual clinical failures? If so, what should the strategy be for patients who fail initial therapy with a quinolone?

L. Peterson: I have three case histories that illustrate treatment failures with quinolones. Until 1996, we had not seen any intermediate or resistant pneumococci to any quinolone, then during 1996, about 10% of our invasive strains were intermediately susceptible to both ciprofloxacin and ofloxacin. In 1997, a patient presented with an acquired immune deficiency not due to HIV. He had chronic pneumonia and had been treated for one month first with azithromycin then ofloxacin and finally developed high fever and looked septic. He was hospitalised with pneumococcal pneumonia that was resistant to macrolides and to ofloxacin. His strain had a single ParC topoisomerase mutation. In 1998, an older female presented with CAP that had been treated unsuccessfully with levofloxacin and she too was a clinical failure. This isolate was resistant to levofloxacin and had two topoisomerase mutations, one each in ParC and ParE. These two patients were sensitive to penicillin and tetracycline, were successfully treated and survived.

Recently, an elderly female patient was hospitalised with bacteraemic pneumococcal pneumonia and meningitis and she died. She had been treated as an outpatient with an intermediate dose of ciprofloxacin for an upper respiratory tract infection. The isolate from this patient was resistant to levofloxacin (MIC 8 µg/mL), ciprofloxacin (MIC 16 µg/mL), sparfloxacin (MIC 8 µg/mL) and trovafloxacin (MIC 4 µg/mL). Moxifloxacin had a MIC value of 2 µg/mL. There are going to be more treatment failures related to susceptibility.

What can we do with outpatients? The new fluoroquinolones may provide the solution. Studies on the efflux mechanism show that a large moiety at the C_7 position on the fluoroquinolone molecule prevents staphylococci and streptococci pumping the drug out of the cell. This is the organisms first line defence. Moxifloxacin and trovafloxacin each have an azabicylo group at C_7 and this prevents the efflux of the drug from the cell. In-vitro experiments have shown that moxifloxacin is less likely to select for mutants than levofloxacin, ofloxacin and ciprofloxacin. If these other quinolones are used in the community, it may result in an increase in the circulation of first-step mutants. This would make it easier to select for second-step mutants, or resistant strains, either in the laboratory or clinically. Thus the new quinolones, such as moxifloxacin and trovafloxacin, could reduce this problem and we should consider using them as first-line therapy in the community.

D. Talan: This leads to the most difficult question. Should there be a quinolone strategy for treating specific infections, designating a certain drug for a certain infection? Should drugs like moxifloxacin be used where they may be best? Are other quinolones better for aerobic Gram-negative infections, like *Pseudomonas*? Should mixed infections be treated with combination therapies to preserve the potency of these drugs?

D. Low: It is an interesting dilemma and a public health issue. There has been ten years experience with ciprofloxacin without much pneumococcal resistance. Maybe part of the reason resistance has not been as prominent is that there are very low inocula in those patients who are colonised. A patient treated for AECB may only have $10^2 - 10^4$ *S. pneumoniae* and the likelihood for a spontaneous resistant mutant arising is low. Now, drugs like levofloxacin are used to treat documented pneumoccocal pneumonias where there may be $10^{12} - 10^{14}$ bacteria in the lungs. The opportunity for a single-step mutant to occur is much greater. It may well be that first-step mutants are already present and, despite having these great new products, it may be too late. Thus we should stop using the older quinolones for community RTI's as soon as possible. There are pneumococci detected in surveillance studies that have MIC values for trovafloxacin of 16 µg/mL.

We should be trying to use these drugs where they are most appropriate. The best example is to treat documented heavy inoculum pneumococcal infections where drugs like moxifloxacin should be first choice.

QUESTION: What do you think about the data that suggests that CAP is a polymicrobial infection, not aerobic nor anaerobic, but atypical that sets up a typical type infection? As empiric therapy, are antimicrobials needed that have activity against atypical as well as typical pathogens?

D. Low: Clinical trials, using monotherapy have not supported it. There is more data that in 5 – 10% of pneumonia there is a co-pathogen, that is two pathogens present. What is needed are clinical trials that compare an agent active against all pathogens with one that is active only against typical pathogens. It is an important question to be answered because it might reduce recovery time.

L. Mandell: Data on 5000 patients in the U.S. showed that those treated according to the ATS guidelines did better than those who were not. The guidelines suggested beta-lactam +/– macrolide. The group with the macrolide did better. So, there is support for the fact that 5 – 16% of pneumonias have co-infections. This retrospective data suggests that there should be coverage for atypical organisms.

There is concern about macrolide resistance and failures but at this time it is perception. Even with penicillin sensitive pneumococcus there are failures. The mortality rate in the first 24 h is the same now as in 1929. We have to keep this in perspective. Every single infection is not cured; a few failures does not mean that certain drugs, as a class, are failing.

QUESTION: General practitioners believe that any quinolone can be used against pneumococcus. Should we designate which of the quinolones are more effective against pneumococcus?

L. Peterson: There are two questions. Because total quinolone use drives resistance to all others in the class, what is the appropriate setting for a quinolone? Once the decision has been made to use a quinolone, the most active one should be used to avoid resistance development. If there is a pathogen involved such as a pneumococcus, trovafloxacin or moxifloxacin should be used. This strategy should retain their usefulness for many years.

CHAPTER 36

Round Table Discussion – Community Issues   36

J. Garau: The new quinolones, especially moxifloxacin, are becoming formidable competitors to agents traditionally used in the treatment of community acquired respiratory tract infections. The key pathogen is the pneumococcus, probably the best example of rapid acquisition of antibiotic resistance. Today, it is not uncommon to have pneumococci resistant to tetracyclines, chloramphenicol, co-trimoxazole, beta-lactams and macrolides. This has become a global problem and the reasons why we are so interested in this new compound. Is there evidence that this increasing prevalence of resistance to these agents later turns into clinical failure?

G. Hoogkamp-Korstanje: The answer is yes and no. Susceptibility or resistance alone does not determine failure or cure. Patients and other factors play a role in determining the outcome of the treatment. There are not many studies that show resistance is the reason for clinical failure. Reviewing these studies, it is possible to see that the higher the MIC value or the higher the MBC (minimum bactericidal concentration), then the risk of failure is higher than the chance of success.

J. Garau: When should we use the new quinolones, such as moxifloxacin, for the treatment of CAP?

T. Marrie: Pneumonia is a complex illness and it has many facets. There are several questions that need addressing, such as, who is admitted to hospital, how long are they given iv antibiotics, how long are they given oral antibiotics and when are they discharged? For the patients that are admitted to hospital, a quinolone, e.g. moxifloxacin, can be used. This has the advantage that one drug is used rather than two. If the patients can eat and drink, they do not need iv antibiotics.

The other question is what is the role for the quinolones to treat outpatients? I was recently involved in a study in which patients were treated as outpatients for pneumonia with either levofloxacin or another antibiotic, usually a macrolide. Patients in the levofloxacin arm tended to have less symptoms at both two and six weeks compared to those treated with the comparator drug. The challenge is to prove whether a quinolone is superior to a macrolide for outpatients.

J. Garau: Could the use of suboptimal quinolones, due either to incorrect dosing or to borderline activity against pneumococcals, endanger susceptibility to moxifloxacin?

C. Nightingale: The probable answer to that question, at this time, is no. The mechanism for the development of resistance requires a two point mutation. The first mutation increases the MIC_{90} value of the bacteria 4–8 fold; the second increases the MIC_{90} value an additional 4–16 fold. If the initial drug is not very active against S. pneumoniae, e. g. its MIC_{90} value is 2 µg/mL, a 4–8 fold increase will take the MIC_{90} value to 16 µg/mL. That probably means the organism is no longer susceptible to the drug and one could predict a high prevalence of failures or lack of eradication of the bacteria.

The question now is what would happen if a patient exposed to that treatment was treated with moxifloxacin. Assume the initial MIC_{90} value for moxifloxacin against the wild type of the organism was 0.12 µg/mL. If there were a 4–8 fold increase due to a first-point mutation, then the MIC_{90} value would be 0.6–1 µg/mL. That concentration is easily achievable using 400 mg doses once a day of moxifloxacin, so it should be able to eradicate the organism. However, as the number of first mutants in the population increases due to older quinolone use, there may be problems for a drug like moxifloxacin.

J. Garau: What factors are driving resistance in the community?

W. Holmes: In the community there are no good diagnostic markers. Physicians refer to treatment failures without having defined what was being treated in the first place. Among patients being treated for lower respiratory tract infections, 15–20 % return with the same symptoms within one month. These patients did not fail to respond to antibiotic; they probably did not have a disease that an antibiotic would treat. Until there are better markers to define illnesses in the community, physicians will contribute to resistance of organisms by poor prescribing.

G. Grassi: Is there evidence that antibiotics may have some benefit in acute bronchitis?

R. Guthrie: That is one of the more difficult questions in primary care. Antibiotics are used regularly and routinely in primary care to treat acute bronchitis. The scientific rationale is limited. Studies do not show success with antibiotic treatment. However, they were small studies which have used older antibiotics such as doxycycline and sulphamethoxazole. Also, the criteria for entry were not well defined, so it is difficult to know what was treated. The patient group could have included viral bronchitis, bacterial bronchitis, allergic rhinitis with cough and bronchospastic disease. The situation in primary care is that antibiotics are regularly used as an empiric treatment with very limited science. There is a need for well defined studies and then an education programme for primary care physicians.